D0989618

Springer Series in Statistics

Statistics in the Health Sciences

Springer Series in Statistics

Anderson: Continuous-Time Markov Chains: An Applications-Oriented Approach.
Anderson/Borgan/Gill/Keiding: Statistical Models Based on Counting Processes.
Andrews/Herzberg: Data: A Collection of Problems from Many Fields for the Student and Research Worker.
Anscombe: Computing in Statistical Science through APL.
Berger: Statistical Decision Theory and Bayesian Analysis, 2nd edition.
Bolfarine/Zacks: Prediction Theory for Finite Populations.
Brémaud: Point Processes and Queues: Martingale Dynamics.
Brockwell/Davis: Time Series: Theory and Methods, 2nd edition.
Choi: ARMA Model Identification.
Daley/Vere-Jones: An Introduction to the Theory of Point Processes.
Dzhaparidze: Parameter Estimation and Hypothesis Testing in Spectral Analysis of Stationary Time Series.
Farrell: Multivariate Calculation.
Fienberg/Hoaglin/Kruskal/Tanur (Eds.): A Statistical Model: Frederick Mosteller's Contributions to Statistics, Science, and Public Policy.
Goodman/Kruskal: Measures of Association for Cross Classifications.
Grandell: Aspects of Risk Theory.
Hall: The Bootstrap and Edgeworth Expansion.
Härdle: Smoothing Techniques: With Implementation in **S**.
Hartigan: Bayes Theory.
Heyer: Theory of Statistical Experiments.
Jolliffe: Principal Component Analysis.
Kotz/Johnson (Eds.): Breakthroughs in Statistics Volume I.
Kotz/Johnson (Eds.): Breakthroughs in Statistics Volume II.
Kres: Statistical Tables for Multivariate Analysis.
Leadbetter/Lindgren/Rootzén: Extremes and Related Properties of Random Sequences and Processes.
Le Cam: Asymptotic Methods in Statistical Decision Theory.
Le Cam/Yang: Asymptotics in Statistics: Some Basic Concepts.
Manoukian: Modern Concepts and Theorems of Mathematical Statistics.
Miller, Jr.: Simultaneous Statistical Inference, 2nd edition.
Mosteller/Wallace: Applied Bayesian and Classical Inference: The Case of *The Federalist Papers.*
Pollard: Convergence of Stochastic Processes.
Pratt/Gibbons: Concepts of Nonparametric Theory.
Read/Cressie: Goodness-of-Fit Statistics for Discrete Multivariate Data.
Reiss: Approximate Distributions of Order Statistics: With Applications to Nonparametric Statistics.
Ross: Nonlinear Estimation.
Sachs: Applied Statistics: A Handbook of Techniques, 2nd edition.

(continued after index)

David S. Salsburg

The Use of Restricted Significance Tests in Clinical Trials

With 24 Figures

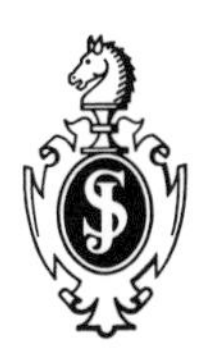

Springer-Verlag
New York Berlin Heidelberg London Paris
Tokyo Hong Kong Barcelona Budapest

David S. Salsburg
Pfizer Research Division
Pfizer, Inc.
Groton, CT 06340
USA

Series Editors

Library of Congress Cataloging-in-Publication Data
Salsburg, David, 1931–
The use of restricted significance tests in clinical trials/by David Salsburg.
p. cm. — (Springer series in statistics. Statistics in the health sciences)
ISBN 0-387-97798-8. — ISBN 3-540-97798-8
1. Clinical trials—Statistical methods. I. Title. II. Series.
[DNLM: 1. Models, Statistical. 2. Probability Theory.
3. Randomized Controlled Trials—methods. 4. Randomized Controlled Trials—statistics. QV 771 S175u]
R853.C55S35 1992
610′.72—dc20 92-2151

Printed on acid-free paper.

Production managed by Francine Sikorski; manufacturing supervised by Jacqui Ashri.
Typeset by Asco Trade Typesetting Ltd., Hong Kong.
Printed and bound by Braun-Brumfield, Inc., Ann Arbor, MI.
Printed in the United States of America.

9 8 7 6 5 4 3 2 1

ISBN 0-387-97798-8 Springer-Verlag New York Berlin Heidelberg
ISBN 3-540-97798-8 Springer-Verlag Berlin Heidelberg New York

Preface

The reader will soon find that this is more than a "how-to-do-it" book. It describes a philosophical approach to the use of statistics in the analysis of clinical trials. I have come gradually to the position described here, but I have not come that way alone. This approach is heavily influenced by my reading the papers of R.A. Fisher, F.S. Anscombe, F. Mosteller, and J. Neyman. But the most important influences have been those of my medical colleagues, who had important real-life medical questions that needed to be answered. Statistical methods depend on abstract mathematical theorems and often complicated algorithms on the computer. But these are only a means to an end, because in the end the statistical techniques we apply to clinical studies have to provide useful answers.

When I was studying martingales and symbolic logic in graduate school, my wife, Fran, had to be left out of the intellectual excitement. But, as she looked on, she kept asking me how is this knowledge useful. That question, what can you do with this? haunted my studies. When I began working in biostatistics, she continued asking me where it was all going, and I had to explain what I was doing in terms of the practical problems that were being addressed.

Throughout human history, there has been a clash between the view that knowledge is a superior good by itself and the view that knowledge should be used to make life better for mankind. The first view was held by the anonymous Talmudic rabbi who denounced those who would learn in order to "have a spade to dig with" and the haughty Plato who compared what little we know to shadows cast on the wall of a cave, while real Truth was too dazzling for ordinary mortals to see. It was Fran who taught me the value of the second view and made me appreciate the efforts of Paul Ehrlich, who wanted to take the abstract knowledge of selective dyes and create "magic bullets" that would cure diseases, or of Benjamin Franklin, whose scientific investigations led to efficient stoves and protection against lightning.

So I dedicate this book to my wife, Francine Thall Salsburg, who made it necessary for me to face the practical consequences that result when we apply abstract mathematical ideas to the problems of human suffering.

Groton, Connecticut David S. Salsburg

Contents

PART ONE

PHILOSOPHICAL AND SCIENTIFIC PROBLEMS WHEN APPLYING STATISTICAL METHODS TO CLINICAL DATA

CHAPTER 1
The Randomized Controlled Clinical Trial

1.1. RCTs as Scientific Experiments

Randomized controlled clinical trials (RCTs) are among the most difficult and expensive of scientific studies. A typical multiclinic study sponsored by a pharmaceutical firm will recruit 200 to 300 patients and cost $1 million to 3 million. A typical multiclinic study sponsored by government agencies like the National Institutes of Health in the United States or the Medical Research Council in the United Kingdom will recruit thousands of patients and cost tens or hundreds of millions of dollars. A study designed to follow patients for 6 months to a year will take 3 to 4 years to recruit enough patients and several more years to analyze the data after the last patient has completed. Not only do RCTs use up large amounts of research money and resources, they also have their costs in the most precious of commodities, human suffering.

These are scientific studies, but that does not define how they should be run or analyzed. Philosophers from Kant to Popper have tried to systematize "scientific method" and establish what it is, but have failed to characterize all of science. This is because science is constantly changing, as new discoveries or new technologies allow for new types of studies. Thus, while the form of the RCT appears to follow that of the typical small-scale pharmacological study in animals, its size and complexity make it something different. And the paradigm of "scientific method" that may be appropriate to animal pharmacology fails to be adequate. In the usual animal study, the experimental units are relatively homogeneous (through the use of inbred strains), the conditions of the study are tightly controlled (for instance, the animals are caged and can be fed fixed rations), and the measured endpoints are few and well defined.

In a human RCT, on the other hand, the subjects are randomly bred and are allowed to wander about eating what they will and engaging in all sorts of disparate activities. In addition, we measure many endpoints. This last is done because cooperative patients are hard to find and we want to learn as much as we can from each one, because we need to follow all sorts of side issues to protect their safety, and because the most precise endpoints that define animal experiments often involve sacrifice of the animals, so we need indirect and usually noninvasive measures for humans. Whereas the animal trial is a small well-focused experiment in which all influences but the treatments are controlled to be the same, the RCT is a large trial in which patients differ considerably from one another, many influences are uncontrolled and often unmeasured, and even the treatments are not always followed exactly.

Add to all of this the facts that patients drop out of RCTs before completing the planned series of visits, that clinic visits occur, at best, at approximately the times planned and that some are missed, and that the measurements that are planned to be taken are seldom taken completely at all visits. What emerges is a complex collection of data filled with random noise, loosely organized around a fiction called the protocol. The first step in the analysis of any RCT is the arrangement of individual patient records to "fit" the protocol. Before we can make any kind of statistical test, we must first decide which record is "baseline," what treatment the patient was on, what visit constituted the "one month" visit, etc. It may turn out that the often arbitrary decisions that organize each patient's record to fit the protocol have a much greater influence on the conclusions of the study than any choice of statistical methodology.

Because of this uncertainty of design and complexity of data collected, it would be a mistake to impose a fixed model of "scientific method," regardless of the pedigree of that model and its usefulness in other fields. Instead, we are better off viewing the results of an RCT as a collection of data accumulated in a somewhat organized way and asking how that data can be used to answer well-defined medical questions. Viewed phenomenologically, the RCT has the following useful aspects:

(1) The patient population is well defined.
(2) Patients are assigned to treatment at random from the pool of eligible patients.
(3) The treatment regimens are well defined, and records are kept of treatments actually used.
(4) Patients are followed intensively across several dimensions.
(5) Endpoints are well defined and documented.
(6) Data are collected and recorded carefully.

In a typical RCT, we locate a group of patients, using consistent and usually objective criteria to define the disease being studied. The patients are by no means a random sample of all such patients. They are patients who are available to the secondary or tertiary treatment centers that take part in the trial and who are willing and able to participate. So, what we have is a group of humans suffering from a particular disease treated with more rigid regimens than would normally be used and followed with a greater intensity of measurement than is usual. From the data that accumulate, we hope to be able to predict what might happen if future patients are treated with similar regimens. We also hope to be able to identify interesting patterns of response in subsets of patients to get a handle on short-term safety problems associated with these regimens, to determine something about the pharmacological response of the human species, and as in all scientific studies, to learn how to design the next study.

1.2. Statistical Considerations

The RCT stands as an exercise in scientific research. It can be thought of as an entity independent of the methods that will be used to analyze the data that emerge. On another level, we can consider a collection of methods of analysis, a sort of mathematical bag of tricks that lets us summarize the data accumulated in these studies. The tricks can range from conceptually simple ones, like computing averages or counting the percentage of patients with specific types of responses, to ones involving heavy mathematical modeling and complex computer programs, like Cox regression or linear-logistic methods. But on a simple level they can all be thought of as a collection of tools, where the only criteria governing their use is whether they enable us to understand the results of the study better.

However, all mathematical tools for data analysis can be derived from abstract mathematical theorems. A typical theorem has a set of assumed hypotheses, a collection of prior theorems to build upon, and a set of conclusions. There is a weak link between the conclusions of a mathematical theorem and the use of a particular tool in data analysis. The tool is "valid" to the extent that its use is compatible with the conclusions of the theorem and the assumed hypotheses hold (or almost hold). These theorems do not emerge out of nowhere. They are suggested by or are part of a large coherent set of theory called a mathematical model. The model is an attempt to describe some aspect of reality in terms of mathematical symbols. So there is an interplay between the mathematical model and the clinical trials that use techniques derived from its theories. With mathematical models, we can embed the analysis of clinical data into the model and determine whether one tool is "better" than another or whether a particular tool is "valid."

This interplay among the RCT, the analysis of its data, and the mathematical model is displayed in Figure 1.1 (derived from Box [1980]). The arrows indicate how information processed in one aspect is applied to another. Note that the mathematical model is subject to change, being influenced by the analysis of data from the clinical trial. Furthermore, the clinical trial is itself

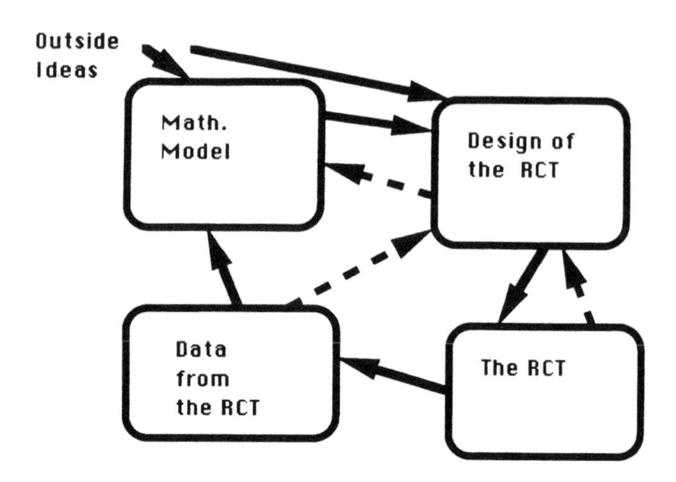

Figure 1.1. Interplay of model, design, and data.

influenced by the mathematical model in the sense that we design the trial to elucidate aspects of the model and we use the model to delineate the limits of the design.

But, beyond the RCT, the analysis of its data, and the theoretical model is something else. This is the philosophical mindset that governs the construction of the mathematical model and its application to the interpretation of the RCT. It is possible to run a clinical trial and interpret the results without using any but the most rudimentary tools of analysis (like averages). It is possible to use mathematical techniques to attempt to make sense out of the data from an RCT without being concerned about a theoretical model. So it is also possible to apply a standard mathematical model while being completely ignorant of the philosophical foundation of the model.

The classic beginning of modern clinical research is the observational study of Pierre Louis on time to recovery for patients who were bled with leeches versus those who were not bled. Louis' analysis consisted of noting that the average time for patients who were bled was greater than the average time for those who were not. This was a clinical trial whose author saw no need to do more than observe and summarize results. The Lanarkshire study (see Gosset [1931]), which compared the overall state of health of children between those assigned an extra ration of milk and those left to the family's usual devices, is an example of a study that used linear regression, a relatively sophisticated tool of analysis, without worrying about a theoretical model. Most modern RCTs are run using a specific mathematical model based on the work of Jerzy Neyman and Egon S. Pearson in the early 1930s (Neyman and Pearson [1928, 1933a, 1933b]), and tools of analysis are judged "appropriate" if they are sanctioned by that model. There have been very lively discussions of the philosophical foundations behind that model in the statistical literature, but one can look in vain in the medical literature for even an acknowledgment that there might be a particular philosophical mindset behind that model.

1.3. The Overall Plan of This Book

This book is designed to examine the three statistical phases of

(1) philosophical foundations,
(2) mathematical models, and
(3) tools of analysis.

Chapter 2 describes the historical development of the Neyman-Pearson model and the criticisms that have been made of it. Chapter 3 discusses the models used by Fisher to develop tools of analysis. Chapter 4 covers a modified model created by Neyman in his later papers and the tools of analysis that come out of that modified model. Chapter 5 discusses the problems in philosophical foundations that arise. Chapters 6 to 12 cover specific tools of analysis that can be derived from Neyman's restricted test model, which I think can prove very useful in the examination of RCTs.

If the reader is interested only in tools, then Chapters 6 to 12 should be the main focus of attention. However, I think that it pays to understand and have a clear picture of one's attitude toward mathematical models and foundations, and I have tried to give the reader sufficient information in the earlier chapters to allow for informed decisions. In fairness to the reader, however, I should make it clear that I have a particular foundational view, which I describe in Chapter 5. This, in turn, leads to a set of recommended procedures when it comes to analyzing data from an RCT, and the descriptions of methods in chapters 6 to 12 are designed to fall within those recommendations. Finally, Chapter 13 contains a fully developed example of the type of statistical analyses proposed in this book.

To avoid misleading the reader, I will summarize my foundational view and recommended procedures here. If these seem so bizarre as to warrant no further exposure, the reader will find it convenient to close the cover at the end of this chapter.

1.3.1. Foundations

Probability has a connection to "real life" only as a measure of the observer's belief. However, psychological studies have shown that most people have incoherent concepts of probability and are consistent only for two levels of probability

(1) Highly improbable (or probable), and
(2) 50:50.

Thus, no matter how exact and sophisticated our calculations of probability can be made, in the end the only calculations that are "useful" are those involving very small (or large) probabilities and probabilities near 50 percent.

1.3.2. Mathematical Models

Because RCTs deal with human responses and a heterogeneous outbred population of subjects, it is impossible to model observed responses exactly. Thus, we have to model responses as consisting of some observable variable, Y, associated with a set of "causative" variables

$$x_1, x_2, \ldots, x_k$$

and some simple function of the x's

$$g(x_1, x_2, \ldots, x_k; \pi)$$

describing how Y occurs "on the average." For any individual patient, the observed value of Y consists of the sum

$$Y = g(x_1, x_2, \ldots, x_k; \pi) + E,$$

where E is the result of all the things we know nothing about, such as the differences between this patient and the "average" patient, the failures to follow protocol, and the lack of compliance. Lacking an ability to put these things into the mathematical model, we call E "random noise."

If we knew the true value of π, then we would not need to observe Y but we could predict the value of Y for every patient after knowing the values of the x's for that patient. The observer has a prior set of beliefs about π that can be described in terms of the range of values that the observer is quite sure π lies within and the range of values that the observer associates with a 50 percent probability of coverage. The data from the RCT is then used to adjust those beliefs, hopefully narrowing the range of possible values of π associated with "quite sure" and "50:50."

1.3.3. The Tools of Analysis

Any attempt to estimate π will prove a waste of time if the random noise in the study is great enough to drown out all signals. A first step in the analysis of any study is the construction of a single well-formulated test of significance that compares the general patterns of outcome across the assigned treatments. Following Neyman's theory of restricted tests, this one overall significance test should be constructed to be most sensitive to the effects that we can reasonably expect to see if the treatments are, in fact, different.

If the overall test of significance fails to produce a p-value that is adequately small to give the observer a personal belief that no difference in effect is highly improbable, then the analysis stops there with a statement that there is no evidence in this study that the treatments differ in effect. This last sentence is stated in the awkward language of significance testing. We examine the case of no effect and conclude that there is an effect if the probability of what we have observed was very small under the assumption of no effect. This resembles the logical technique known as *reductio ad absurdum*, where we assume the condition we wish to disprove and show that it leads to a logical contradiction. However, as will be shown in Chapter 3, the connection is logically faulty.

If the overall test of significance produces a small enough p-value, then we have a license to hunt. Using the mathematical model as a guide, we formulate medically sensible questions we might pose of the data and determine ranges of answers about which we are "quite sure" and ranges of answers about which we associate a 50 percent probability.

Chapters 6 to 12 describe methods of deriving very sensitive overall tests of significance that can be applied to RCTs. Even if the reader does not buy into my whole foundation-model-analysis structure, the restricted tests described in these chapters may be of use within other structures.

CHAPTER 2

Probability Models and Clinical Medicine

2.1. What Is Probability?

The mathematical theories of probability start with an abstract "space" of "events." The events in the space can be combined according to the rules of set theory.

Probability is defined as a measure imposed on the events in the space. The link between this abstract space with probability measuring its events and what we observe in a scientific study is a "random variable." A random variable is a means of turning events in the space into observable numbers.

As a simple example, we might roll a pair of dice and record the sum of the numbers that appear on top when they stop. The space of events is the set of all possible pairs of numbers from the dice. The random variable is the sum of the faces. If we distinguish between the two dice, each event has probability of 1/36, but the probability associated with specific values of the random variable is not so simple. If we record a sum of 6, it could have resulted from any of the following pairs of numbers (events):

$$(1, 5), (5, 1), (2, 4), (4, 2), (3, 3).$$

So the probability of getting a sum of 6 for our random variable is $5 \times 1/36$ or 0.13888 ....

In real life, this mathematical idea of a space of events and a random variable is a useful tool, but the identification of the underlying space of events is not always very clear. Suppose we run an RCT and find that 50 percent of the patients exposed to treatment A and 40 percent of the patients exposed to treatment B responded. Let the random variable be the difference in response rate

$$Y = 0.50 - 0.40.$$

When it comes to using probability theory to deal with scientific experiments, where is the space of events with probability measuring the events from which the random variable is derived?

Gosset (who achieved immortality under the pseudonym Student and discovered the distribution of Student's t-statistic) said that the space of events was the set of all possible studies that might have occurred. Fisher (the founder of modern mathematical statistical theory) suggested, in one paper, that the space was the set of all possible permutations of patient assignments to treatment that might have occurred. This is a slightly smaller set than Gosset's set of all possible things that might have occurred. But both are flawed because they postulate a space of things that did not happen (and could not happen since the study we observed is the one that did occur). Furthermore, Gosset's approach does not tell us how to compute the probabilities associated with random variables on the space of all possible events.

Earlier in the century, Pearson introduced some of the now-standard tools of statistics from a different point of view. Pearson was the intellectual heir of Sir Francis Galton. Along with Galton, he was one of the founders of the pioneering journal, *Biometrika*, whose purpose, according to the initial publication notice, was to use statistical models to show the minute changes in species due to natural selection that might occur within a human lifespan. In Pearson's formulation, the statistician starts with a large number of individuals in a given species and measures some common item in all of them, such as cranial capacity in skulls taken from ancient graves or beak lengths in a particular species of tropical bird. Since the statistician cannot collect all the members of that species, this large collection has to serve as a representative sample. From that sample, Pearson tried to determine the true frequency distribution associated with all members of that species. He proposed that we could compare the frequency distributions of different species of or the same species from different environments and show examples of evolution as subtle shifts in the parameters of the best fitting models.

Pearson followed this approach because he was building on theoretical work he had published in the late 1890s. In his theoretical papers, Pearson started with the central limit theorem:

If we have a large number of independent random variables,

$$W_1, W_2, W_3, \ldots, W_n$$

which represent "errors" or small individual deviations from some norm, then the sum of those errors

$$X = W_1 + W_2 + \cdots + W_n$$

has a Gaussian or normal distribution (*the famous "bell-shaped curve"*).

In Pearson's formulation, we measure some variable Y on a given individual from a species. Biology can be thought of as a mathematical function that converts an underlying characteristic, X, which is the sum of a large number of "errors," into an observable measurement, Y.

$$Y = f(X) \quad \text{for some unknown function } f(\ ).$$

If the function $f(\ )$ is sufficiently smooth, it can be approximated by a third-degree polynomial (using Taylor's theorem). Using that approximation and calculus to derive the probability distribution of Y, if X has a normal distribution, Pearson derived a family of probabilities known as the Pearson family of skew distributions. Any particular skew distribution is described uniquely by four parameters:

(1) the mean,
(2) the variance,
(3) the skewness, and
(4) the kurtosis.

Pearson hoped to show the effects of evolution in terms of these four parameters.

2.2. The First Use of Significance Tests by Pearson

The early issues of *Biometrika* were devoted, for the most part, to collecting large amounts of data from correspondents and finding the skew distributions that fit that data. Early on, Pearson discovered a simple tool for determining if a given skew distribution fit the data. Figure 2.1 shows the frequency curve for a skew distribution broken up into eight regions, each of which has a probability if 0.125. If there are N observations and if this distribution fits the data, we would expect each region to contain

$$0.125\ N$$

observations. But this is a random sample of the set of all data, so it is not unexpected that we might have slightly more or slightly less in each region. Pearson reasoned that the occurances of an observation in a given region is relatively rare (a 12.5 percent chance), so the count of such observations should follow a Poisson distribution. This implies that the mean of the number of observations is the same as the variance, so that

$$\text{mean} = 0.125\ N \quad \text{and} \quad \text{variance} = .125\ N.$$

If the mean is 5 or greater, then the Poisson distribution is approximately normal, so

$$(\text{Observed } \# \ -0.125N)/\surd(0.125\ N)$$

has a standard normal distribution with mean = 0 and variance = 1.

Since Pearson was interested in detecting differences from the expected that were either too large or too small, he squared this standardized variate

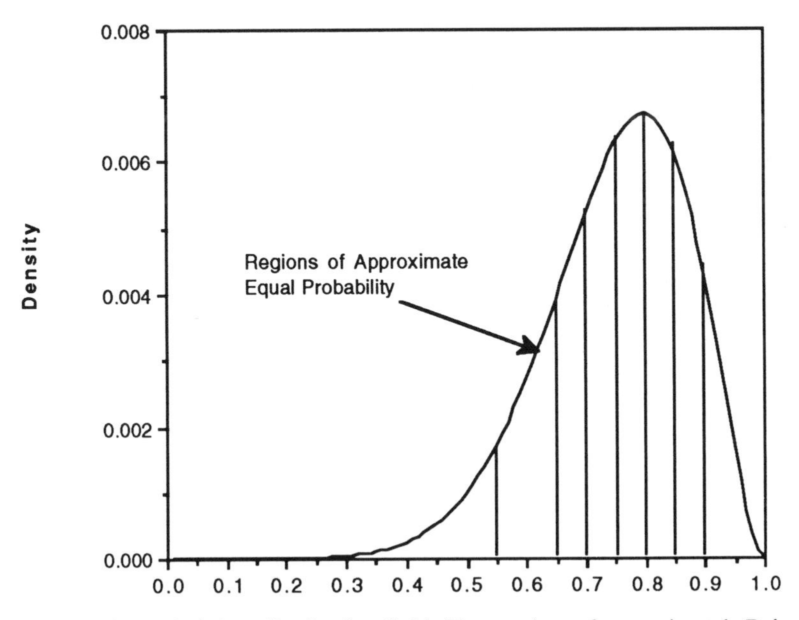

Figure 2.1. Theoretical skew distribution divided into regions of approximately Poisson probability.

and added the squared variates for each region

$$\chi^2 = \sum (O_i - 0.125\ N)^2/0.125\ N,$$

where O_i = number observed in the ith region and χ is the Greek letter chi. Pearson showed that its distribution belonged to his family of skew distributions and tabulated the probabilities associated with large values of χ^2. This use of a computed test statistic to check on the validity of a mathematical assumption about the probability distribution of data was not original to Pearson. Attempts had been made in the late 19th century to determine whether the stars in the heavens were randomly distributed. But Pearson's chi-square became the first systematic use of significance testing to aid in interpreting random data (see Fisher [1937]).

2.3. Fisher's Contribution

Fisher (who single-handedly developed most of what is now taught in first-year courses in mathematical statistics) took Pearson's idea of a test statistic and refined it. Fisher started with agricultural experiments at Rathhampstead Experimental Station in England. The story of how he reorganized the nature of agricultural experiments belongs elsewhere. But by the

AJAX	K OF K	NITHSDALE	GREAT SCOTT	DUKE OF YORK
GREAT SCOTT	DUKE OF YORK	ARRAN COMRADE	IRON DUKE	EPICURE
IRON DUKE	EPICURE	AJAX	K OF K	NITHSDALE
K OF K	NITHSDALE	GREAT SCOTT	DUKE OF YORK	ARRAN COMRADE
	UP TO DATE	KERR'S PINK	UP TO DATE	BRITISH QUEEN
	BRITISH QUEEN	TINWALD PERFECTION	EPICURE	KERR'S PINK
	KERRS PINK	UP TO DATE	IRON DUKE	AJAX
	TINWALD PERFECTION	ARRAN COMRADE	BRITISH QUEEN	TINWALD PERFECTION

Figure 2.2. Layout of treatments in blocks of soil from one of Fisher's early papers.

middle 1920s, Fisher had established basic principles of experimental design, which included methods of statistical analysis. In Fisher's formulation, the experimenter started with a mathematical model that described the type of effect he or she (some of Fisher's best collaborators at that time were women) expected to see from applying a treatment to soil or the plants. The experimental field was divided up into small blocks in such a way that each block tended to have the same level of "fertility." Each block was then further divided into small plots (holding 10 to 20 plants). (See Figure 2.2.) The treatments to be tested were randomly assigned to plots within blocks. The experiment ran, and the grain was harvested from the interior plants of each plot.

The weights of grain from each (block)X(plot) were small and did not differ much from one another. As an example, let

$$X_{1j} = \text{weight of grain from treatment 1 in block } j,$$

$$X_{2j} = \text{weight of grain from treatment 2 in block } j,$$

$$X_{1.} = \text{average weight from treatment 1 across all blocks,}$$

$$X_{2.} = \text{average weight from treatment 2 across all blocks.}$$

Since $X_{1.}$ and $X_{2.}$ are sums of small independent random variables, they have a Gaussian or normal distribution (remember the central limit theorem?). All Fisher needed was a decent estimate of their variance and he could determine if the difference was more than might be expected by chance alone. The random assignment of treatments to plots within blocks gave him a tool that allowed for estimation of the variance of each observation X_{ij}. If he was careful in balancing the experiment and if the measurement was appropriate, then the variance would be the same across all plots and blocks. So Fisher got an estimate of variance that was made more precise by his use of all the data, and he could use the fact that

$$\mathrm{Var}(X_{i\cdot}) = \text{underlying variance}/n, \quad \text{where } n = \text{number of blocks}$$

to determine whether the observed averages, $X_{1\cdot}$ and $X_{2\cdot}$, differ by more than might be expected by chance. Other experimenters tried to "improve" on Fisher's method by assigning treatments to plots within the blocks according to elaborate patterns, designed to minimize the variability between measurements. Fisher [1926] rejected these procedures. He pointed out that the act of randomly assigning treatments to plots guaranteed that the variance estimate would be unbiased. The systematic assignments produced variance estimates that were biased downward, so that use of them would produce "significant" findings when the mean difference between $X_{1\cdot}$ and $X_{2\cdot}$ was, in fact, within the range that might be expected from chance alone.

At this point, the double (and sometimes contradictory) reasons for random assignment of treatment to plot come out. The usual reason given for random assignment of patients to treatment in a randomized controlled trial is that it "balances" the treatments with respect to the many uncontrollable (and often unmeasured) factors that might influence patient response. To this end, it is traditional to display the relative assignment to treatment in terms of sex, race, age, and baseline measurements of disease when writing a report on an RCT. Furthermore, there is a strong opinion in the medical community that a study that turns out to be unbalanced with respect to a key variable should be taken with a grain or salt. In Fisher's formulation, the "balance" that results from randomization is a beneficial side effect. The main purpose of randomization is to allow for unbiased estimation of variance. If, ex post hoc, it turns out that the "balance" was not perfect, it does not affect the validity of the statistical calculations.

Eventually, Fisher developed general procedures for the analysis of data from a designed trial. These procedures are described in a "cookbook" he wrote, *Statistical Methods for Research Workers* (Fisher [1970]), which went through many editions. The successive editions served to correct minor errors (both typographical and mathematical) and to respond to critics. There are no mathematical derivations in *Statistical Methods* and very little philosophical discussion. The reader is told to do this or that and given numerical examples to show how. However, once in a while the idea behind significance testing emerges, along with Fisher's general view of its usefulness:

> In preparing this table we have borne in mind that in practice we do not want to know the exact value of P for any observed chi squared, but, in the first place, whether or not the observed value is open to suspicion. If P is between 0.1 and 0.9 there is certainly no reason to suspect the hypothesis tested. If it is below 0.02 it is strongly indicated that the hypothesis fails to account for the whole of the facts. We shall not often be astray if we draw a conventional line at 0.05, and consider that higher values of chi-square indicate a real discrepancy.

Note that he does not say what to do if the p-value is between 0.1 and 0.05.

In the rest of the book, Fisher applies significance testing to data from randomized experiments, but he does not address the rationale again. What emerges from a review of all of Fisher's published papers is that Fisher treated significance testing as a rough and ready tool, whose rationale ran something like this:

> We have used several treatments in an experiment. We do not expect the effects of the treatments to be the same, but we would like to know whether the study provides useful information. So we set up a straw-man, the hypothesis that the treatments have the same underlying mean effect. We compute a test statistic whose probability distribution we can calculate under this null hypothesis. If the value of the test statistic is improbably large, then we have evidence that the data from this study emerged from something other than the null hypothesis.

In his agricultural papers, Fisher would often examine the data and construct his test statistic from the most extreme differences he found.

Fisher's view of what this significance test meant appeared in a paper (Fisher [1929]), where he justified the use of statistical significance tests to debunk experiments in psychical research:

> It is a common practice to judge a result significant, if it is of such a magnitude that it would have been produced by chance not more frequently than once in twenty trials. This is an arbitrary, but convenient, level of significance for the practical investigator, but it does not mean that he allows himself to be deceived once in every twenty experiments. The test of significance only tells him what to ignore, namely all experiments in which significant results are not obtained. He should only claim that a phenomenon is experimentally demonstrable when he knows how to design an experiment so that it will rarely fail to give a significant result ....

Gosset ("Student") wrote something similar at about the same time (Gossett [1931]):

> This inability to detect abnormalities extraneous to the test itself is shared by all single tests of significance and the result is that the wise man will never go further in the direction of asserting similarity than to say, "The sample affords no evidence that, etc."

However, for both men, the formulation of significance testing rested on poor philosophical grounds. The probability space that generated the random variables and allowed for calculation of significance tests consisted of a vague collection of events that "could have happened." Furthermore, there were often several competing test statistics that could be computed from the data. Which one should be used?

2.4. The Neyman–Pearson Formulation

In 1929 Egon Pearson, the son of Karl Pearson, raised this question to Jerzy Neyman, a young Polish mathematician: When we test whether data are normally distributed, how do we know that the tests we have chosen are adequate to the question if they all turn out to be nonsignificant? Karl Pearson had treated the chi-square test of goodness of fit as proof that a given frequency distribution did fit the data. He would find the general member of his class of skew distributions that seemed to fit and then refine the estimates of the parameters so as to minimize the chi-square test statistic.

Neyman, at that time, was a mathematician and had little or no experience with biological data. His sense of mathematical correctness was disturbed as he learned about significance testing. Two things bothered him. One was the lack of a solid description of the "space" of "events" that generated the probability.

To Neyman, the only justification for applying probability to real-life problems lay in the law of large numbers. If we claim that the probability of tossing two dice and getting a sum of 6 is 5/36, then we can toss two dice thousands and thousands of times, and the long-run proportion of times we get a sum of six will become arbitrarily close to 5/36. This is the frequentist interpretation of probability, and Neyman was a frequentist. Thus, for significance testing to make sense to Neyman it had to be justified on frequentist grounds.

The other problem with significance testing that Neyman saw is illustrated by Figure 2.3.

Suppose we have observed a normally distributed random variable and found that

$$X = 0.$$

We wish to test the null hypothesis that X is distributed normally with mean 0 and variance 1. The probability that the observed X will exactly equal zero is as small as we want to make it. This is because the probability of observing a value of X in some region is the area under the normal frequency curve about that region. So we can construct a very small region around 0. It will contain the value of X, but its probability will be very small. Thus, having a small probability for an observed test statistic is not enough reason to reject the null hypothesis.

Neyman solved the second problem by postulating more than the null hypothesis. Fisher saw the null hypothesis as a straw-man, which was most

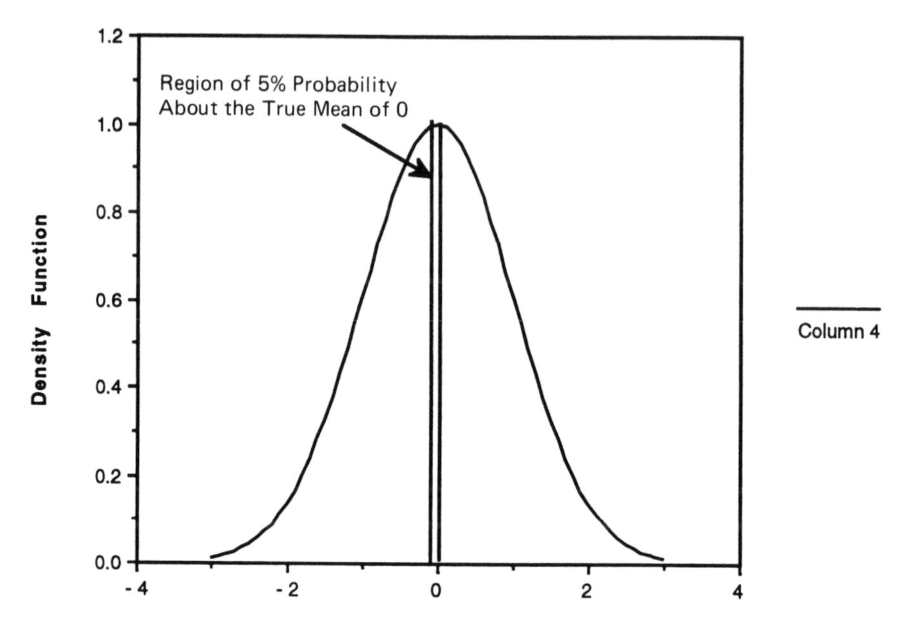

Figure 2.3. Example of a foolish "rejection" region for testing the null hypothesis that the data are distributed normal (0, 1).

likely not true and was used as a tool for determining if the study had enough information in it to allow the analyst to estimate what was true. Neyman saw that the only way to justify rejecting the null hypothesis for a large value of the test statistic was by having an alternative hypothesis, which would produce large values of the test statistic if it were true.

Once he postulated two hypotheses, the null and an alternative, Neyman conceived of the experimenter as engaging in a long string of experiments and making a decision after each one. It was Fisher's view that the null hypothesis was merely a straw-man and that one could only reject it since a nonsignificant test statistic did not imply that it was true. However, Neyman formulated the problem so that the decision is whether to accept the null hypothesis or the alternative hypothesis. This leads to the two-way table illustrated in Figure 2.4., which can be found in most elementary statistics textbooks. Neyman formulated the problem as one in which the experimenter wishes to minimize the number of times he or she will make a mistake. Since there are two types of mistakes possible:

Type I, the experimenter says H1 is true when H0 is true
Type II, the experimenter says H0 is true when H1 is true,

there are two probabilities of error

$$\alpha = \text{Prob}\{\text{type I error}\},$$

$$\beta = \text{Prob}\{\text{type II error}\}.$$

True State of Nature

DECISION TAKEN	H0 is True	H1 is True
Decide H0 is True	no error	Type II Error
Decide H1 is True	Type I Error	no error

Figure 2.4. Interplay of model, design, and data.

Under Neyman's frequentist interpretation, these probabilities are, in fact, the proportion of times the experimenter will make mistakes in this long run of experiments.

Once the problem had been formulated this way, it was possible to derive theorems and lemmas about the relative relationships of the two hypotheses and the alpha and beta levels. This, of course, is the type of neat mathematics that appeals to writers of textbooks and is relatively easy to teach.

Having formulated the problem in traditional mathematical terms, Neyman and Pearson now set out to optimize. That is, they began to examine methods of statistical analysis that would be "best" in some sense. After all, Pearson's original question was how he might know what the "best" test of normality was. Unfortunately, the problem has three variables

(1) α, the probability of a type I error;
(2) β, the probability of a type II error; and
(3) δ, the "distance" between the null and alternative hypotheses;

and α and β have an inverse relationship. Decreasing one means increasing the other. The problem had to be further reduced to allow for optimization. Although none of these appear in the Neyman–Pearson correspondence, it is not hard to propose several possible formulations:

For a given region of values for δ, minimize $\alpha + \beta$.
For all δ, minimize $\alpha \times \beta$.
Fix α and β and minimize δ.

Since the null hypothesis is often easy to formulate and since for many alternative hypotheses the probability distributions may be difficult or impossible to compute, Neyman and Pearson chose the formulation: Fix α and minimize β for all δ. This is the "uniformly most powerful" test or set. To tear apart the words,

$$\text{"power"} = 1 - \beta.$$

If we pick a particular value of δ, an α-level "most powerful" test is one that has a fixed value of α and greater power against an alternative hypothesis defined by δ than any other test.

"Uniformly most powerful" means most powerful over all possible values of δ.

This was a very neat summing up of the problem. By the 1940s. Abraham Wald had extended the basic ideas to a general mathematical formulation called "decision theory." In the early 1950s, Erich Lehmann (Neyman had moved to the United States and founded the mathematical statistics department at University of California, Berkeley, and Lehmann was one of his fellow faculty members) published a widely influential book (Lehmann [1959]) in which he enlarged upon the Neyman-Pearson formulation of hypothesis testing and defined new criteria for

uniformly most powerful unbiased tests,
uniformly most powerful invariant tests,
least favorable priors,
etc.

These further developments of Lehmann were needed because, early in their investigations, Neyman and Pearson had discovered that, in Neyman's words (Neyman [1935b]):

> Unhappily, uniformly most powerful sets occur very infrequently. In fact, the set that is most powerful for one hypothesis H1 may even be less powerful than alpha for another hypothesis H2.

One situation where uniformly most powerful tests cannot be constructed occurs when we are comparing the incidence of a particular event (like cardiovascular death) between two treatment groups and the hypotheses are

$$\text{H0}: p_1 = p_2, \quad \text{where } p_i = \text{probability of event for treatment } i,$$

$$\text{H1}: p_1 \neq p_2.$$

This, of course, is one of the most widely occurring comparisons in the analysis of RCTs. Thus, the Neyman–Pearson formulation, for all its neatness, is theoretically inappropriate for many RCTs.

Neyman himself, as he accumulated experience in statistical analysis, never returned to the Neyman–Pearson formulation. His last published article on the subject is a review of the results for a French journal in 1935, in which the pessimistic phrase quoted just appeared. When his colleague Erich Lehmann prepared his elaborate mathematical extension of the Neyman–Pearson formulation, Neyman seemed uninterested according to some members of the faculty with whom I have spoken.

But through the rest of his career, Neyman did pursue one aspect of this early work. He continued to look at the consequences of defining the alternative hypotheses very carefully. One result was a series of lectures on what he called the restricted chi-square tests (Neyman [1949]; Fix, Hodges, and Lehmann [1959]).

The next chapter will deal with Fisher's criticisms of the Neyman–Pearson formulation. The chapter after that will attempt to meld Fisher's approach to significance testing (as articulated in his criticisms) and Neyman's insights about alternative hypotheses.

CHAPTER 3

Significance Tests Versus Hypothesis Tests

3.1. Fisher's Views of the Neyman–Pearson Formulation

Ronald Aylmer Fisher, the man who developed the concept of significance tests applied to randomized controlled experiments, greeted the Neyman–Pearson formulation of hypothesis testing with scorn. When Wald expanded the ideas into a more general decision theory, Fisher was even more vehement in his denunciations (Fisher [1955, 1959]). His basic criticism of the Neyman–Pearson formulation appeared in a letter to the editor in *Nature* in the early 1930s (Fisher [1935]):

> For the logical fallacy of believing that a hypothesis has been proved to be true, merely because it is not contradicted by the available facts, has no more right to insinuate itself in statistical than in other kinds of scientific reasoning. Yet it does so only too frequently. Indeed, the "error of accepting an hypothesis when it is false" has been specially named by some writers, "errors of the second kind." It would, therefore, add greatly to the clarity with which the tests of significance are regarded if it were generally understood that tests of significance, when used accurately, are capable of rejecting or invalidating hypotheses, in so far as they are contradicted by the data; but that they are never capable of establishing them as certainly true. In fact that "errors of the second kind" are committed only by those who misunderstand the nature and application of tests of significance.

By 1955, Fisher had formulated a theory of significance testing to compete with Neyman–Pearson, which he published first as an article in the *Journal of the Royal Statistical Society* [1955] and then, more elaborately, as a book [1959]. Unfortunately for the argument between Fisher and Neyman, it was one-sided. Neyman did not respond with written articles and made no attempt to defend either the Neyman–Pearson formulation or its more general version, decision theory. I met with Neyman a few years before he died and asked him about this dispute. He put off any discussion of this dispute as something that involved Fisher's irascibility and that he did not consider important. The personalities of the two were quite different, Fisher always spoiling for a fight and quick to respond to fancied injuries of his *amour propre*, and Neyman, ever the gentleman, kind and available to students and careful never to hurt anyone's feelings. However, my reading of Neyman's papers suggests to me that he agreed in principle with most of Fisher's criticisms and tried to gently direct statistical methodology along other lines—in particular along lines suggested by the use of restricted tests, which will be discussed in the next chapter.

Fisher's basic criticism of the Neyman–Pearson hypothesis testing formulation was that it did not reflect what was actually done in scientific research. He distinguished between scientific research and "acceptance procedures" (Fisher [1959]):

> Now, acceptance procedures are of great importance in the modern world. When a large concern like the Royal Navy receives material from an engineering firm it is, I suppose, subjected to sufficiently careful inspection and testing to reduce the frequency of acceptance of faulty or defective consignments. The instructions to the Officers carrying out the tests must also, I conceive, be intended to keep low both the cost of testing and the frequency of the rejection of satisfactory lots. ... the logical differences between such an operation and the work of scientific discovery by physical or biological experimentation seem to me so wide that the analogy between them is not helpful....

With this, Fisher dismissed Neyman's frequentist interpretation of the probability of a false significance. Instead, Fisher concentrated on what he called "inductive reasoning," the use of observational data to build mathematical models. He pointed out that all the standard tests of significance (most of which he himself had invented) were based on conditional probabilities. That is, some of the events that occur in a scientific experiment are ancillary to the main measurement. If we wish to estimate the slope of a linear regression, the intercept of the regression line is ancillary to our search. These ancillary events are random, but we act as if they were fixed at their observed values and compute probabilities conditional upon those fixed values. In this sense, no experiment is ever repeatable exactly, and Neyman's frequentist interpretation of the significance test has no meaning.

For the scientific experimenter to engage in "inductive reasoning," Fisher claimed there had to be four conditions. Two of them are quite obscure and refer to Fisher's (unstated) philosophy of probability. But the other two are quite relevant to the analysis of RCTs. One is that there has to be a rich multiparameter mathematical description of the probability distribution that is used to describe the random fall of the data. This mathematical description allows us to use the data to reject some versions of the model. The second requirement is that we use all the data. In Fisher's words, "inductive reasoning is more strict than is deductive reasoning, since in the latter any item of data may be ignored and valid inferences may be drawn from the rest; i.e. from any selected subset of the set of axioms used, whereas in inductive inference the whole of the data must be taken into account. ... The political principle that anything can be proved by statistics arises from the practice of presenting only a selected subset of the data available" (Fisher [1959]).

3.2. Problems with the Frequentist Definition of Probability

In the meantime, Neyman–Pearson hypothesis testing and the frequentist interpretation of probability were falling on bad ways. There is one fundamental problem with the Neyman–Pearson formulation. The optimization requires that the alpha level be fixed in advance (usually at 0.05). Doing this results in a type I long-run error rate of 5 percent. But, the only decisions that can be made are that H0 is true or that H1 is true, regardless of the computed p-value. If $p = 0.04$, the decision is that H1 is true. If $p = 0.004$, the same decision is made. If $p = 10^{-10}$, the same decision is made. The decision is also independent of the mean difference between treatments, so a treatment that produces a 20 percent increase over placebo results in a decision that is equivalent to one where the treatment produces a 120 percent increase over placebo. There is no such thing in Neyman–Pearson hypothesis testing as "almost significant" or "highly significant." There is no place in the Neyman–Pearson formulations for a less-than-certain decision. We must decide on either H0 or H1.

Some of the deepest thinkers in probability theory, A. Birnbaum, J. Kiefer, and K. Arrow, tried to find reformulations of Neyman–Pearson that allowed for more complex decisions. And each one showed that a more complex conclusion cannot be supported by the frequentist theory of probability (Berger [1983]).

Along another line, in 1956, Savage and Bahadur hacked a hole in the basic foundation of significance/hypothesis testing (Bahadur and Savage [1956]). They considered the following situation. We have a test statistic, T, and a null hypothesis that the expected average value of T is some number μ_0. The alternative hypothesis is that the expected value of T is $\mu_1 \neq \mu_0$. We can set μ_1 as far away from μ_0 as we wish, but we can still find a distribution of T, which has an expected value μ_1 but for which the probability of finding T significantly far from μ_0 is less than alpha. That is, if we allow the class of alternative distributions to be "big" enough, then there is no way of detecting a mean difference, no matter how large, with any power.

The Savage–Bahadur distributions, the class of alternatives that cannot be distinguished from the null hypothesis, are mixtures of two distributions. One part is far from the null. The other part is far on the other side. See Figure

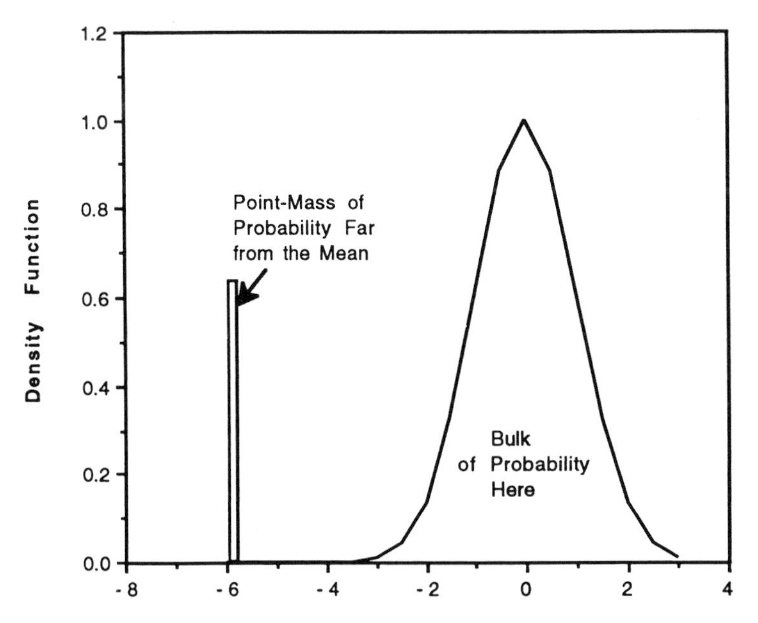

Figure 3.1. Example of a Savage–Bahadur distribution.

3.1 for a schematic description. It is possible to approximate a Savage–Bahadur distribution in a real-life RCT. Suppose we have a disease where the test treatment can vastly improve conditions for some patients but cause others patients to deteriorate. For instance, patients in congestive heart failure often have inappropriate cardiac responses to natural hormones as part of the way in which their bodies have reached homeostasis. If we give an adenergic blocking agent to congestive heart failure patients, we might upset this precarious homeostasis on some patients but improve the condition for those in whom the aspect being blocked is aggravating their condition. The average response across all treated patients will be the same as the average response across the placebo patients, but specific subsets will show dramatic differences.

The Savage–Bahadur paper is really an extension of one of Neyman's original insights. We need to define alternative hypotheses in order to test for significance, said Neyman. He then showed that the optimum solution (uniformly most powerful tests) seldom existed, if we allow the class of alternatives to be too wide. As an even worse conclusion, Savage and Bahadur showed that no testing is possible if we allow the class of alternatives to be too wide. None of these findings is related to the frequentist definition of probability. They arise from abstract mathematical manipulations of the theories of probability and are independent of what we really mean by probability.

Thus, by the early 1960s, the philosophical foundations of the Neyman–Pearson formulation lay in shambles. Fisher had shown that the formulation was inappropriate for scientific research, Kiefer and Arrow had shown that there was a fundamental inconsistency that could not be done away with, and Savage and Bahadur had shown that use of "standard methods" can lead to serious errors. However, the Neyman–Pearson formulation had made its way into elementary statistics textbooks as the only formulation. These same textbooks failed to recognize the need for restriction of the alternative hypotheses and taught a brand of statistical analysis that was at best useless and at worst detrimental to the development of scientific knowledge. It was this inappropriate formulation that made its way into the medical textbooks and has come to dominate the methods of analysis applied to randomized controlled trials in the medical literature.

3.3. Significance Testing Versus Hypothesis Testing

There have always been voices criticizing Neyman-Pearson in the statistical literature. The most prominent have been Box [1980], Anscombe [1957, 1963], and Barnard [1985], all of them English statisticians who had learned from Fisher or Fisher's students. In 1977, David Cox, another English statistician, tried to revive Fisher's ideas of significance testing in a more modern framework. Cox noted that significance tests were being widely used in scientific research, and he examined the ways in which they were applied.

Cox divided the use of significance tests into two types. In one type we wish to refine a mathematical model, what he calls the use of "plausible null hypotheses." The other he called "dividing hypotheses." When using dividing hypotheses, we wish to distinguish between two competing models. Significance tests are used in developing plausible nulls in a way similar to the way Karl Pearson used the chi-squared test to refine his parameter estimates. The analyst has a model with many parameters and uses significance tests to find a parsimonious model that fits the data as well as more complicated models. When using dividing hypotheses, we postulate two distinctly different models and use significance tests to distinguish which one fits the data better or whether neither fits the data well.

A major component of the criticisms of the English school is that scientific research is not a series of identical or nearly identical studies, as in the case of acceptance sampling (viz. Fisher). Instead, we create an interaction among experiments, data analysis, and models, refining each new experiment to take advantage of insights gained and constantly revisiting the data from previous experiments in the light of new results and newly proposed models. Figure 3.2 (which appeared in Chapter 1) displays this schematically and is taken from Box. Philosophically, the English school continues to follow Fisher, using significance tests as a relatively vague and rough cutting tool, where there is no particular predetermined level of significance that signifies action or nonaction.

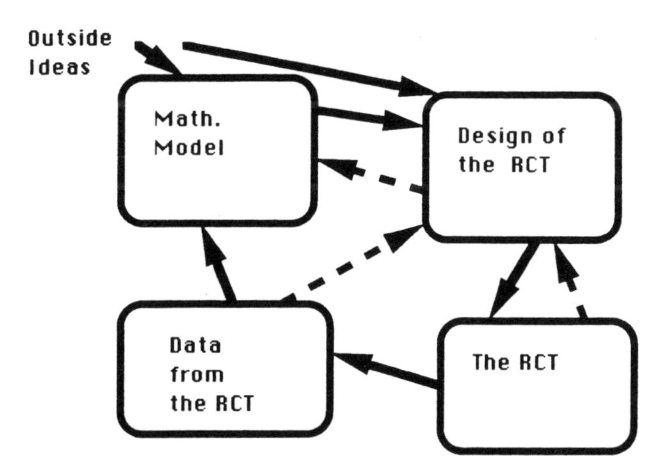

Figure 3.2. Interplay of model, design, and data.

3.4. Philosophical Problems

All the preceding describe how one goes about using the calculated p-value of a significance test to examine the results of a study. But the calculations are based upon probability theory, and the philosophical problem of identifying the mathematical concept of probability with "real life" remains unresolved. It is fairly clear that despite the efforts of excellent mathematicians like Neyman, Arrow, Kiefer, and Birnbaum, the frequentist interpretation is a dead end that cannot be used to justify the many subtle ways in which the scientific community has found significance testing useful.

A full discussion of the various definitions of probability and the relationships between probability and inductive reasoning can be found in Cohen [1989]. Cohen points out that we can think of probability as referring to observable events or propositions about events. The frequentist interpretation applies only to the probability of observable events. However, inductive reasoning can use probability calculations only if they result in probabilities about propositions. Cohen provides meta-mathematical proofs that there is no direct connection between probability statements about A, conditional on B, and the logical statement that B implies A.

We can put Cohen's criticism in the framework of significance testing by considering the simple situation of a lottery with N tickets, where each ticket sells for one dollar and the winner takes all N dollars. Suppose we try to link significance testing to inductive reasoning by equating the following statements:

I. Probability of an event under the null hypothesis is very small, therefore we reject the null hypothesis.
II. The null hypothesis is not true.

If N, the number of tickets in the lottery, is very large, then the event

Ticket Number 1 will win the lottery

has low probability. This holds for the events

Ticket Number 2 will win the lottery
Ticket Number 3 will win the lottery
Etc.

We now equate events and hypotheses, so we can reject the null hypothesis

Ticket Number i will win the lottery

for any particular value of i. If we say this is the same as the logical deduction that ticket number i will not will the lottery, then the rules of logic tell us that the union of false propositions is false, and we can conclude that no ticket will win the lottery.

Cohen's solution to the problem that probability statements cannot be made equivalent to logical statements is to reject probability statements entirely and describe inductive reasoning in terms of modal logic. Much earlier, John Maynard Keynes (of economic theory fame) proved the same theorems (Keynes [1921]) and concluded that the inductive scientist needs to accompany any probability calculation with a set of weights associated with observable evidence, where those weights have to be derived independently of the probability calculations.

A less abstract discussion of the various interpretations of probability can be found in Shafer [1990], but the same general conclusions appear: (1) The frequentist interpretation is philosophically flawed, and (2) it is necessary to bring something else into the discussion to go from probability values to inductive reasoning.

In 1985 Lawrence Brown presented what should be the final blow to the frequentist interpretation of probability in the prestigious Wald Memorial Lectures. He was building on earlier work by Cox [1958]. We can put Brown's paradox within the setting of a clinical study by considering a study with a measurable outcome that defines efficacy (such as a decrease in diastolic blood pressure), along with some other random event that occurs during the course of the study. The second random event need not be directly related to the outcome variable. In fact, In Cox's version of the paradox, the second random event is the actual numbers of patients who are enrolled in each treatment group (as opposed to the planned number). Using statistical decision theory, the optimum statistical procedure for dealing with the efficacy variable can be computed for each possible outcome of the unrelated random event. Yet, if we average across all possible outcomes of the random event, then none of these optimum procedures is optimum for the average. This is the paradox.

In a clinical setting, the paradox says that if we find formal "significance" for the outcomes of this particular study, it may be completely irrelevant to what might happen when these treatments are applied to a larger more general patient population. Suppose, for instance, that the study at hand used a peculiar set of patients whose genetic characteristics produce an unusual response to treatment. If this were known, then the medical community would hesitate to extrapolate the results to a more general population. Such an extreme case is clear, but the Brown lectures show that the failure to extrapolate can hold for much more subtle differences between the current study and the "outside world." The "outside world" is the average across all possible configurations of the ancillary random event. The results of the study are restricted to the particular outcome that has been observed.

Brown then shows that there is only one way around this paradox. The only solution is a Bayesian one. We must enter with some prior belief about the probability of outcomes for the patients in the "outside world" and use the results of this study to modify those prior beliefs. Only by use of this prior probability distribution can we produce methods of analysis that both hold for the peculiar events of this study and are extrapolative to a more general class of patients.

3.4.1. Salvaging Neyman's Insights

Neyman based much of his theoretical work on the frequentist interpretation of probability. But the failure of this interpretation does not mean that all his work must be discarded. The formal structure of hypothesis testing (with its foundation on a fixed probability of a false positive) cannot hold up, but many of Neyman's ideas can be adapted to a less severe definition of probability. In the next chapter, I will examine Neyman's later work, which I believe provides a useful set of tools for the analysis of RCTs, allowing us to improve upon the English school's roughly defined concept of significance testing. I will address Brown's paradox in Chapter 11.

CHAPTER 4
Neyman's Insights

Jerzy Neyman's contributions to mathematical statistics did not stop with the Neyman–Pearson formulation of hypothesis testing. He was an imaginative prolific thinker who lived into his late eighties. In addition to founding the Department of Statistics at the University of California, Berkeley, he organized a series of seminal conferences (The Berkeley Symposia on Mathematical Statistics and Probability), he encouraged and developed a generation of students who have made their mark on the subject, and he continued to turn out original papers that are a delight to study and that contain strikingly original contributions.

Two of these contributions are particularly relevant to the analysis of randomized controlled trials. These are the concepts of restricted tests and of confidence intervals.

4.1. Restricted Tests

As indicated earlier, an important insight Neyman brought to his early work with Egon Pearson was the realization that one cannot test whether data fit a null hypothesis without having an alternative hypothesis against which to compare it. Savage and Bahadur expanded that insight by showing that the set of alternative hypotheses cannot be allowed to be too large. By the early 1960s, Neyman had refined this into the realization that the narrower the class of alternatives, the greater the possible power.

In some sense, we can think of a significance test as a measure of the "distance" from the observed data to the hypothesis being tested. Figure 4.1 illustrates this. In Figure 4.1, the large triangle represents the set of all

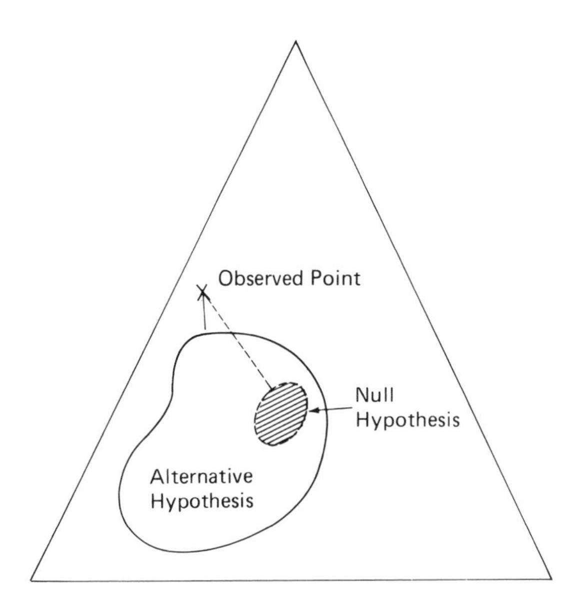

Figure 4.1. Schema of null and alternative hypotheses.

possible hypotheses, the large unshaded figure is the set of alternative hypotheses, the smaller shaded figure (located inside the larger figure) is the set of null hypotheses, and the point denoted "X" represents the observed data.

[My mathematical training forces me to be more specific about this figure. What follows inside these brackets is a careful definition of the meaning of symbols in Figure 4.1. Those who feel the need for mathematical rigor may want to read it. Those who are willing to work with relatively vague analogies may skip to the end of this paragraph. The RCT produces a set of data, which can be thought of as a multidimensional vector. The data, however, have some sort of structure, so subsets of the data can be lumped into groups, and we can count how many observations fall in each group. This collection of groups can be described in terms of the probability of finding an observation in a given group. The triangle represents the simplex of all such probabilities. All these probabilities lie between zero and one and all mutually exclusive probabilities must sum 1.0. A given hypothesis is defined by a point in the simplex, and a class of hypotheses by a region in the simplex. The observed data are the realization of a specific hypothesis, the hypothesis that attributes a probability to each group that is equal to the proportion of data found in that group. The simplex is thus a space of hypotheses, formulated as vectors of probabilities. It has nothing to do with Gosset's vague space of all possible "events." It is a well-defined mathematical object.]

The null hypothesis is nested within the class of alternative hypotheses. For instance, we might have patients exposed to placebo and three different doses of an antihypertensive. Suppose we observe the percentage of patients

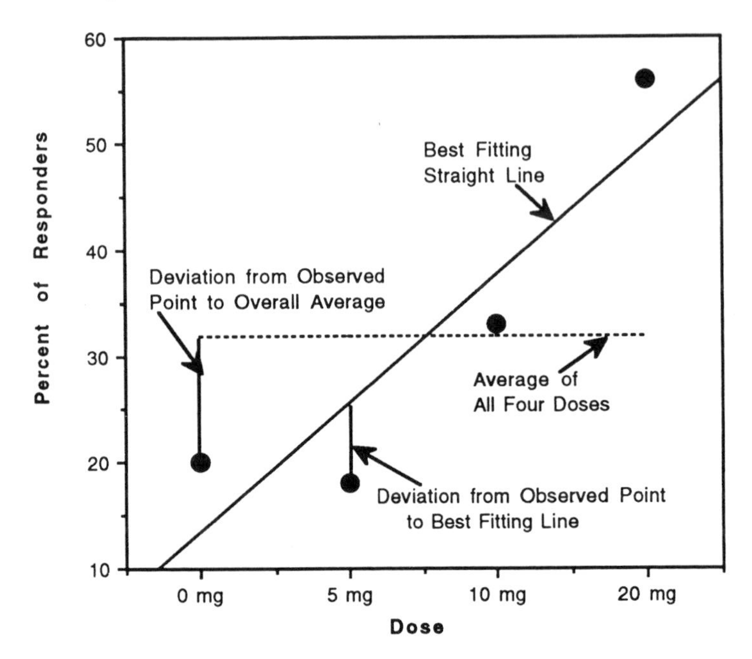

Figure 4.2. Example of dose response where alternative hypothesis is modeled. Percent of responders = A + B (dose).

who "respond" (by some clear-cut definition) within 3 weeks. Figure 4.2 shows a hypothetical plot of such data. For the class of alternatives, consider the model

$$\text{Prob}\{\text{Response}\} = p_0 + \text{B} \times \text{dose}.$$

If the treatment has no effect, then we would expect that all treatments (including placebo) have the same probability of response. So the null hypothesis can be described as the subclass of models where

$$\text{B} = 0.$$

Although it is usually hidden in the computational formulas, most significance tests are nothing but a comparison between the distance from the observed point to the nearest point in the set of null hypotheses and the distance from the observed point to the nearest point in the larger set of alternative hypotheses. In the example shown in Figure 4.2, we first act as if the null hypothesis was true (B = 0) and estimate p_0 as the average proportion of response across all four treatments. The sum of the squared deviations from the observed proportions to that average is the "distance" from the data to the null hypothesis. Next, we fit a straight line by least squares to get a best estimate of both p_0 and B together. We take the sum of the squared deviations between the predicted proportions and the observed proportions as the "dis-

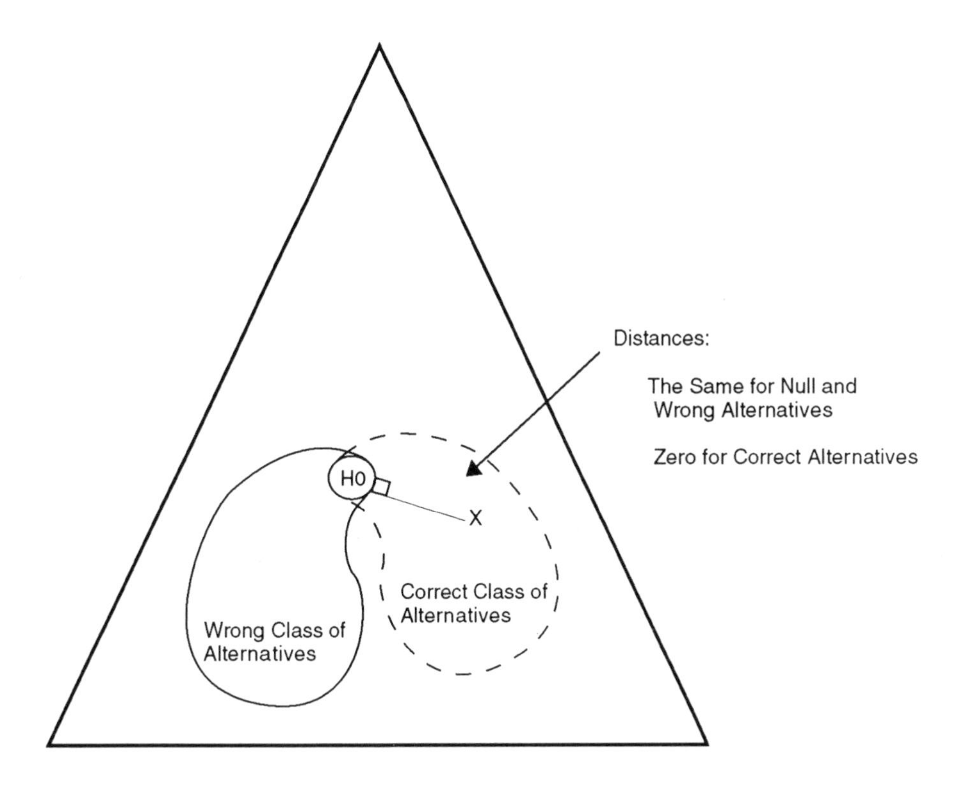

Figure 4.3. Schematic representation of different alternative hypotheses.

tance" to the nearest point in the class of alternative hypotheses. The standard F-test for regression is the ratio of these two "distances."

The data in Figure 4.2 illustrate an essential weakness of this approach. The statistical test carries with it a class of alternatives that is implicit in the computations. But this implicit class of alternatives may not be an appropriate class for the data that emerge from this trial. Figure 4.3 displays a simplex in which there are two regions of alternative hypotheses. The observed point is far from the null, but it is also far from the nearest point in one of the regions of alternatives. It is much closer (in fact, is within) the other region of alternatives. So if the first region is the appropriate class of alternatives, there is no "significant" evidence against the null. If the second region is appropriate, there is "significant" evidence against the null.

Although the highest dose of drug produces a twofold increase in percentage of responders in Figure 4.2, the test for slope does not come out significant. This is because the data do not fit a straight line very well and the deviations about the best fitting straight line are almost as great as the deviations about a constant. Suppose we know enough about the pharmacology of this drug to suggest that one or more of the doses was well below an effective threshold for most patients but that the highest dose was picked to have a clear-cut pharmacological response. Then we would not expect the probability of response to increase linearly (or even steadily) across all doses. Bartholomew has a test of dose response, where the class of alternatives is larger than the set of linear response (Barlow, Bartholomew, Bremner, and Brunk [1972]). Bartholomew's test considers all possible monotone responses (where $\text{dose}(i) < \text{dose}(i + 1)$ implies $p(i) \leq p(i + 1)$). This includes all linear dose responses, all constant "dose responses" (the null hypothesis), but also all responses with plateaus. For the data displayed in Figure 4.2, Bartholomew's test shows a high degree of significance.

Neyman's insights have, thus, two branches. We can improve the power of a significance test if we restrict attention to a small class of alternatives. But we can destroy the power of a significance test if we choose a test that is designed to be powerful against the wrong class of alternatives. This does not mean that a test against the wrong class of alternatives will not find significance. The data may be so far from the null hypothesis that almost any test will show significance. But, if that happens, the *pro forma* test of significance becomes a mere invocation to the gods of publication. The fact that very few RCTs produce such clear-cut results is one of the reasons for writing this book.

This brings me to a major theme of this book. The "standard" significance tests (analysis of variance, t-tests, Fisher's exact test, etc.) all are restricted tests against classes of alternatives that can be described. In most cases these classes of alternatives are inappropriate to the medical or pharmacological reality of the study. The proper analysis of an RCT starts with a well-developed biological model of what might be expected and uses significance tests that are tailored to alternative hypotheses generated by the biological model. When the major tool of the statistician was the desk calculator, it was not possible to run significance tests so carefully tailored, and we had to do with tests that could be run by calculating sums and sums of squares. Most computer packages use these calculator-based algorithms and restrict analysis to the classic "standard" tests. But the modern computer is capable of far more, and we should not be bound to what was convenient to an analyst in the 1930s. In Chapters 6 to 11, I will investigate classes of alternatives that are appropriate for many RCTs and the significance tests associated with them.

4.2. Confidence Intervals

Fisher and the English school (including Box, Barnard, Anscombe, and Cox) treat significance tests as rough cutting tools. We can also use significance tests to sketch in the class of models that appears to be appropriate. However, Fisher contributed more than significance testing methodology. One of his major contributions was to organize a theory of statistical estimation. For instance, once we are reasonably sure that the data can be described in terms of a linear dose response, we will want to know the slope of that response. Or, once we are convinced that treatment A is associated with a lower incidence of MIs than treatment B, we would like to know how much lower.

So the estimation of parameters represents a fine-tuning of the general sketch of models that come from significance testing.

Fisher laid down some criteria for point estimates, that is, for estimates that consist of specific numbers. He defined the concepts of consistency, bias, and efficiency. He then provided methods of estimation that produced "good" estimates. But, the researcher needs to know more than a point estimate. The experiment carries a "smear" of uncertainty due to random noise, and a range of estimates can better convey the information that lies within the data than a single value.

Fisher had some ideas for producing a range of estimates, but so did Neyman. The starting point for both was the fact that the mathematical formula for the density function of the normal distribution,

$$\frac{1}{\sqrt{2\pi}} e^{-\frac{1}{2}(x-\mu)^2},$$

has two symbols:

$$x = \text{the variable} \quad \text{and} \quad \mu = \text{the underlying mean parameter},$$

which are logical duals. That is, the formula looks the same if x were replaced and μ and μ by x. Thus, the formula could be looked upon as describing a density in x or as describing what Fisher called a "fiducial distribution" in μ. If one drew the density function as a function of μ for a fixed observed value of x, as in Figure 4.4, then the middle 90 percent region would describe a range of estimates of μ that are supported by the data.

Fisher tried to extend this by looking at other frequency formulas as functions of the parameters and tried in several papers to elucidate this concept of "fiducial distributions." The effort died with Fisher.

Neyman, on the other hand, saw that the endpoints of this interval of estimates could be calculated by plugging different values of μ into the significance tests and finding those values that just barely showed formal "significance." In this way, values of μ less than the lower bound and greater than the upper bound would represent null hypotheses that would have been rejected by the data. For every parameter in a model there is a test statistic whose computation involves entering a value of that parameter (as the null hypothesis), so Neyman reasoned we could find ranges of parameter values that would not be rejected, and those ranges would represent a "smear" of uncertainty associated with the parameter estimation.

The "smear" of uncertainty has several useful properties. It gives us a reasonable set of values that can be used in predicting future events. And

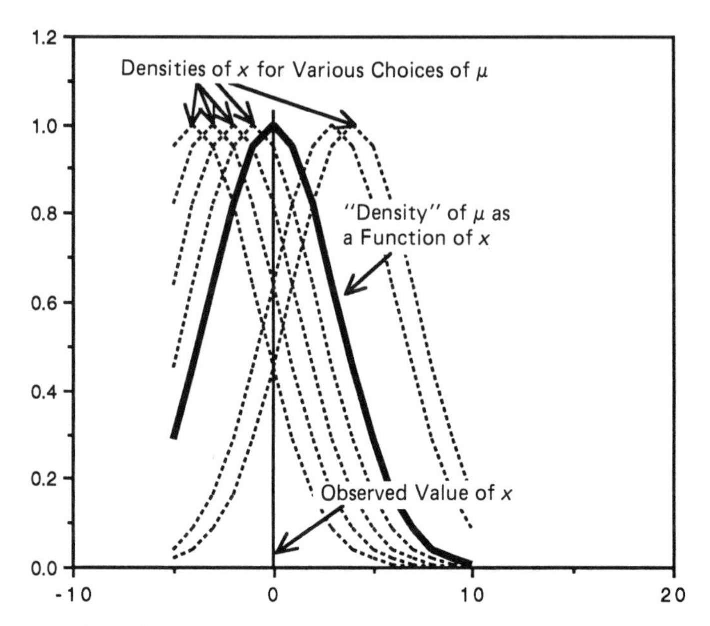

Figure 4.4. Fisher's fiducial intervals: Densities of x versus "density" as a function of μ for fixed x.

its width is a measure of the quality of the study. If there are too few patients, the interval is wide. If there are "enough" patients but the results are highly variable, the interval is wide. If there are enough patients and there is little variability, the interval is narrow. The distance from the endpoints of the interval estimate to the original null hypothesis allows us to distinguish between different types of results, solving the problem that Birnbaum, Kiefer, and Arrow showed could not be solved within the framework of frequentist probability theory.

4.3. The Meaning of Probability, Again

But, having a method for calculating ranges of estimation is not enough. What does this activity mean? If we pick 5 percent rejection regions, does it mean that we are "95 percent sure" that the true parameter lies within the interval estimated? If so, what does it mean to say "95 percent sure"? And the problem comes back to the meaning of a mathematical calculation involving probability, when it is applied to real-life situations.

Neyman proposed a solution, in his first paper describing what he called "confidence intervals" (Neyman [1934]). [It is interesting to note that at the meeting of the Royal Society at which this first paper was presented, one of the commentators objected to the word "confidence" because he foresaw that someone would interpret it as meaning we are "95 percent confident" that the true mean is in the interval. Neyman responded by pointing out that he purposely chose the word "confidence" to avoid confusing it with probability and that no one would be expected to make such an obvious logical error.] Neyman's first solution was completely out of keeping with Neyman's reputation as a frequentist.

He proposed that the true value of the parameter, call it μ, has a probability distribution, that for the various experimental setups, Nature will present us with different values of μ. This is known, in statistical parlance, as a Bayesian position. The Bayesian statistician postulates an unobservable probability distribution for the parameter and treats the observed random variable and the parameter as having a joint probability distribution. Within a Bayesian framework, significance tests make no sense but the analyst can discuss the probability that the parameter lies in a given region. However, Neyman was not interested in the complete Bayesian solution. He was only interested in creating a mathematical gimmick that allowed him to provide a meaning for the coverage of a confidence interval.

He said, let us denote Nature's (unknown) probability distribution for μ as a frequency function

$$\rho(\mu).$$

Suppose we can construct our confidence interval on μ by considering an interval on the observed random variable, X, such that the probability of that interval is at a fixed level, say 0.95. This probability describes the way in which future values of X would fall, as a function of the unknown parameter, μ. He called this the probability of coverage. We can now calculate the average probability of coverage across all possible values of μ,

$$\int L(x, \mu)\rho(\mu)d\mu,$$

where

$L(x, \mu)$ is the probability of coverage for x and μ.

Since $L(x, \mu)$ is constant (always set at 0.95, for instance), this constant value comes out of the integral sign and the average probability of coverage is

$$L\int \rho(\mu)d\mu = L,$$

because the integral of any frequency function is always 1.0.

In other words, whatever meaning we associate with probability in real life, the probability of having μ inside the confidence interval is 0.95 on the average, over all possible values that μ might take on. This does not mean that the probability of coverage is 0.95 for a particular experiment. It only means that this procedure, used over and over, will provide us with an average coverage of 0.95 across many experiments. Note that, unlike the Neyman–Pearson formulation, these need not be a long run of identical experiments.

Neyman's proof of average coverage holds for more than some unknown Bayesian prior distribution on the parameter, μ. The same proof goes through if the probability distribution deals with random subsets of the patients. That is, we can compute a confidence interval on some parameter for a subset of the patients, identified after examination of the data, and we can say that the average coverage is as stated. Suppose, for instance, that we wish to know how long it takes for a hypertensive to have its effects, if it is going to have an effect. We can take the patients who "respond" by some criteria and run a confidence interval on the average time to "response." That confidence interval can then be used to answer the medical question posed. Neyman's method of providing a smear of uncertainty can be applied *ex post hoc* to conclusions derived from exploratory data analysis.

Neyman got into trouble on two counts from his proposal for the computation of confidence intervals. Fisher accused him of "rediscovering" fiducial intervals, and in his later published works Fisher never seemed to understand how Neyman's confidence intervals differed from his own formulation, although it is difficult, if not impossible, to determine how Fisher derived fiducial intervals in complicated multiparameter situations, while Neyman's method is quite simple and straightforward.

Neyman's second problem arose when an American visiting student, Churchill Eisenhart, accused him of mathematical sleight of hand. The prior distribution on μ, which I designated $\rho(\mu)$, appears in the proof and then disappears without ever having played a role in the computation. Furthermore, Neyman's derivation begs the question of what the probability of coverage means. It merely allows us to calculate a probability according to the mathematical rules. It doesn't tell us what that means in real life. Under prodding, Neyman reconsidered the matter and then showed that using the same rules for computation one could view the confidence interval from a given experiment as a random interval (Neyman [1935b]). Using a frequentist interpretation of probability, we can then say that, in the long run, 95 percent of the confidence intervals will cover the true value (which is assumed to be the same for all experiments).

This is the interpretation that is taught in most elementary statistics courses. However, the exact link between probability theory and real life has never been established and the frequentist position is not necessarily an appropriate one. So I prefer to let the mathematical manipulations continue to produce statements about probability and leave the meaning of those statements for personal interpretation. Neyman's first formulation does just that.

In the previous chapter, I looked at the English school's rough formulation of significance testing, as contrasted to the neat (but inappropriate to most scientific investigations) Neyman–Pearson formulation. In this chapter, I examined insights from Neyman's later papers. In the next chapter, I will show how to combine these two approaches.

CHAPTER 5
Reconciling Fisher and Neyman

5.1. What Has Been Developed So Far

The major themes of the previous chapters are

(1) The randomized controlled clinical trial is a complex scientific experiment that is expensive to run and that yields a rich lode of data.
(2) Probability calculations can be made from data, but there is no satisfactory way of relating those probabilities to real life.
(3) Significance testing, as developed by Fisher, is a relatively vague tool, in which probabilities are calculated as a means of rejecting null hypotheses, which are postulated as straw-men.
(4) Significance tests must be directed against a well-defined class of alternative hypotheses that represent what is really expected to happen, and the narrower the class of alternatives, the more powerful the test.
(5) Confidence intervals can be calculated through the use of the algorithms of significance tests, but they can be applied to randomly chosen subsets of the data without invoking the problems associated with significance tests applied to subsets of patients.

This sets the stage for an approach to the statistical analyses of randomized controlled clinical trials that can make use of the insights of both Fisher and Neyman.

5.2. The RCT as an Experiment in Medical Science

Since an RCT is an experiment in the field of medical science, it should start with a set of clearly stated medical questions rather than with a statistical method or model. Asking whether the mean change in standing systolic blood pressure is greater on altenolol than it is on placebo is a statistical question, not a medical question. Asking whether patients on clofibrate have a reduced probability of fatal Ml is not specific enough to be a useful medical question. I believe that useful medical questions are those whose answers enable a practicing physician to treat a specific patient. There is also a class of medical/economic questions that ask about the relative cost and benefit of different treatments. To be able to answer these types of questions, we have to scrub the discussion clean of the pseudostatistical questions that have cluttered the statistical analysis of most RCTs and get back to the science.

Here are a few medical or medical/economic questions that seem to be important.

—Is there an identifiable subset of patients in whom treatment A will "work" or will prove intolerable?
—If treatment A is going to "work," what can be measured to show whether it is working in a given patient, and how long should the patient be followed?
—What is the average number of days of hospitalization using treatment A versus using treatment B?
—What is the average extension of life gained by use of treatment A versus use of treatment B?
—What percentage of patients will have a major extension of life span with treatment A versus treatment B?
—What are the average number of days of work lost with treatment A versus treatment B?

What characterizes all these questions is that they require careful examination of the details of data accumulated in an RCT. Such a careful examination includes a certain amount of exploratory data analysis, such as identification of interesting subsets of patients or comparison of outcomes among "responders" and "nonresponders."

But one major statistical problem holds back such a detailed analysis of data. What if all the differences we see are due to purely random noise? What if there is no difference between treatment A and treatment B and we end up chasing Anscombe's [1985] Will 'o the Wisps. This question was phrased slightly differently by Fisher. Is the experiment worth examining? Fisher's answer was to first run a significance test. If the computed p-value is large, we state that the experiment is one we can ignore, since it does not appear possible to disentangle the relative effects of the comparative treatments from random noise. The choice of a p-value that defines "large" should be left to the situation. If the study is extremely difficult to run (for instance, involving a rare disease), we may be willing to risk a p-value cutoff as high as 0.10. If the study is one of a number addressing the same question and there is already an accumulation of data, then we might require a p-value of 0.01 or less before spending the effort in detailed analysis.

Thus, my proposal is that we first run a formal significance test, using all the patients and all the data. Let

$$X_A = \text{the primary measure of efficacy for treatment A,}$$

$$X_B = \text{the primary measure of efficacy for treatment B,}$$

then the null hypothesis (straw-man) to be tested is

H0: the probability distribution of X_A is the same as the probability distribution of X_B.

[Note that this is not the usual "null hypothesis" used in the analysis of RCTs. The null hypothesis usually tested is that the underlying means of X_A and X_B are the same. For reasons that will be clear when I deal with paradoxical findings, it makes sense to use this more general null.]

Using Neyman's insights, we construct this significance test to be most powerful against a small class of reasonable alternatives. That is, using medical and pharmacological knowledge, we construct scenarios of what we would expect to see if there were difference in this measure between the two treatment groups. Those scenarios are used to form mathematical descriptions of alternative hypotheses.

For instance, we might be comparing an antibody to the toxins of septic shock versus placebo. Patients can be categorized in terms of severity of illness at baseline. Those who have a mild level of morbidity can be expected to recover relatively rapidly on placebo, and any relative improvement will be small. Those with severe morbidity and several symptoms may have already suffered organ damage, and they can be expected to have a high death rate on both treatments. Those with moderate morbidity will probably show the greatest difference in response. Then it seems reasonable to categorize the patients by baseline severity and to construct alternative hypotheses where the probability of death, given treatment, has a pattern somewhat like that in Figure 5.1.

Once a picture like Figure 5.1 is constructed, we can set up mathematical models that approximate such a result, including one or more parameters which that define the null hypothesis when set to zero. This is not an unheard-of process. When considering linear dose responses, we let the alternative hypothesis be that the underlying mean value of some random variable, Y, be such that

$$E(Y) = A + B \times \text{dose}.$$

The null hypothesis of no dose response is equivalent to the null hypothesis that $B = 0$.

The use of a tight class of alternative hypotheses based on what would be expected if a true difference between treatment existed provides two advantages. As Neyman has shown, the power to detect a difference is increased, so a failure to find significance can be taken as fairly strong evidence that this study can provide no information about any difference between treatments.

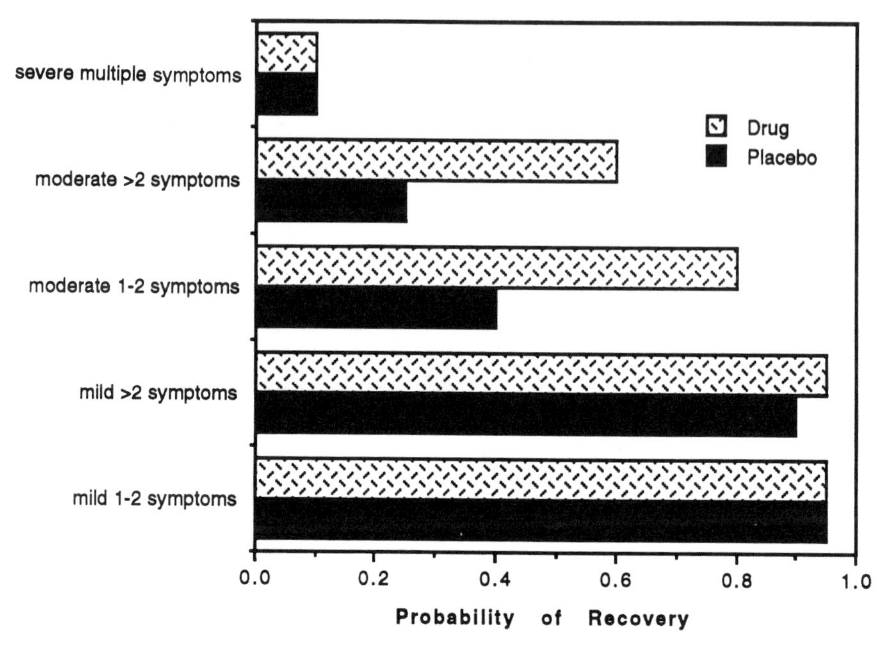

Figure 5.1. Probability of recovery by baseline severity for patients with toxic shock.

A second advantage is that the parameters of the alternative model (and any subgrouping that was used) can answer specific medical or medical/economic questions, so the detailed data analysis that follows a finding of "significance" will be derived from the characteristics of the data that lead to a low *p*-value.

If a medical question has a numerical answer, then that answer can be written, in mathematical terms, as a functional on the family of probability distributions. That is, the answer can be symbolized with a mathematical formula that requires us to know the true probability distribution of the random variables being used. Of course, we don't know that true distribution, but the development of mathematical statistics over the past 70 years has been dominated by methods of estimation that use data-driven approximations of that distribution.

At one time, many of these methods appeared to be different in structure. However, Bradley Efron [1982] has shown that they are, in fact, all based on the empirical probability distribution, the ordered listing of the data observed. Efron has produced a computer-intensive technique, the bootstrap, for estimating the answer to a medical question as a function of the empirical distribution function. When the parameter being estimated is one of those investigated in the past (such as the mean of a normal variate), the bootstrap reduces to the standard method. For such situations, the standard algorithms are much faster than the bootstrap. But computing power has become so fast and inexpensive that this is not an important consideration.

So with the modern computer, there are no longer any limitations on what we can estimate. If the question has a numerical answer and there is no obvious standard method of answering it, the bootstrap will do. Furthermore, the bootstrap can also be adopted to produce confidence intervals on that answer (Efron [1987]). The analyst and the medical community are not bound to the use of standard statistical methods like linear models, logistic regression, analysis of variance, *t*-tests, or Fisher's exact test. One of these standard tools may, in fact, be an appropriate one, but that should be determined only after a well-defined medical question has been posed.

Thus, the third part of my proposed methodology: After a significance is found, we should construct confidence intervals on the answers to a set of medical or medical/economic questions. These may involve subsets of patients or interrelationships among response variables or unexpected "glitches" in the data. Neyman's first formulation of confidence intervals provides a rationale for constructing confidence intervals conditional on random aspects of the data.

5.3. Probability as a Measure of Belief

This brings us back to a fundamental philosophical problem. What does a coverage of 95 percent or of 80 percent for a confidence interval mean? We have finessed the question of what the *p*-value means by treating it as a rough tool for deciding whether or not to examine the data from a study in detail. But we cannot be so cavalier about confidence interval converage. This is because we may get different endpoints to the confidence interval if we use 80 percent coverage or 99 percent coverage. We should have generally accepted rules to guide the choice of coverage.

What is probability when it refers to real life? Birnbaum, Kiefer, and Arrow have shown that the frequentist interpretation is useless when it comes to describing how probabilities are used in scientific research. There is another school, usually associated with Savage (of Savage-Bahadur in a previous chapter), which claims that probability is a personal measure of belief (Savage [1954, 1961]). Each person evaluates statements in terms of how true he or she believes that statement to be. This personal measure of belief is the probability that that statement is true. Cohen [1989] claims that the personal probability definition is the only one that is potentially useful for inductive reasoning.

The first use of the word "probability" occurs in Bernoulli's *Ars Conjecturi* and is used to describe a degree of personal belief (see. Shafer [1990]). So it would appear that the personal definition of probability is not only a useful one but probably the only useful one. The concept of personal probability has been investigated in psychology, and a large number of experiments have been run to elucidate numerical values from individuals.

The experiments have been disappointing for the most part. See Kahneman, Slovic, and Tversky [1982] for a description of many of these experiments. Most people do not carry a coherent set of personal probabilities. That is, if an experimental subject in one of these studies indicates that A is less probable than B and that B is less probable than C, it does not always turn out that the same person believes that A is less probable than C. Furthermore, it is difficult to get people to express their personal probabilities as numbers. No one can really distinguish between events whose probability is 0.67 and those whose probability is 0.76. So at first glance the concept of personal probability would appear to be as useless as the frequentist interpretation.

[Some psychological studies of personal probability have made use of sophisticated betting schemes, where the subject is given a choice of different monetary payoffs subject to different conditions that allow the experimenter to determine results about which the subject is indifferent. These can be converted to probabilities or relative odds. But even these studies show a lack of coherence for many subjects, and broad ranges of indifference indicate that most cannot make fine-tuned decisions.]

However, what has emerged from these studies is that most people are consistent in their ability to understand the difference between extreme probabilities and a probability of 1/2. When given a sequence of events, subjects can distinguish between those sequences that involve extreme probabilities and those that occur with a 50:50 chance. And faced with examples most people can consistently classify events in the categories

very low (or very high) probability, and
50:50 chance.

More sophisticated thinkers, like practicing scientists, can often distinguish another level of probability, something that is better than 50:50 but not particularly sure. So, for those who would make use of the findings of RCTs, we can act as if there are at most three distinguishable levels of probability:

very low (or very high),
50:50, and
something in between.

This matches the results one gets when computing the endpoints of confidence intervals. Figure 5.2 graphs the endpoints of confidence intervals on the mean of a normal variate (with variance = 1.0). The graph rises most rapidly for coverage greater than 90 percent, so a choice anywhere in the range 60 percent to 80 percent produces a similar endpoint. This is true for confidence intervals on other parameters. It is not really necessary to define an exact level to approximate the personal probability concept of "something in between." For purposes of calculation, let us fix on 75 percent coverage.

Thus, the confidence intervals that are computed to cover the numerical answers to medical or medical/economic questions can be put into three categories of coverage:

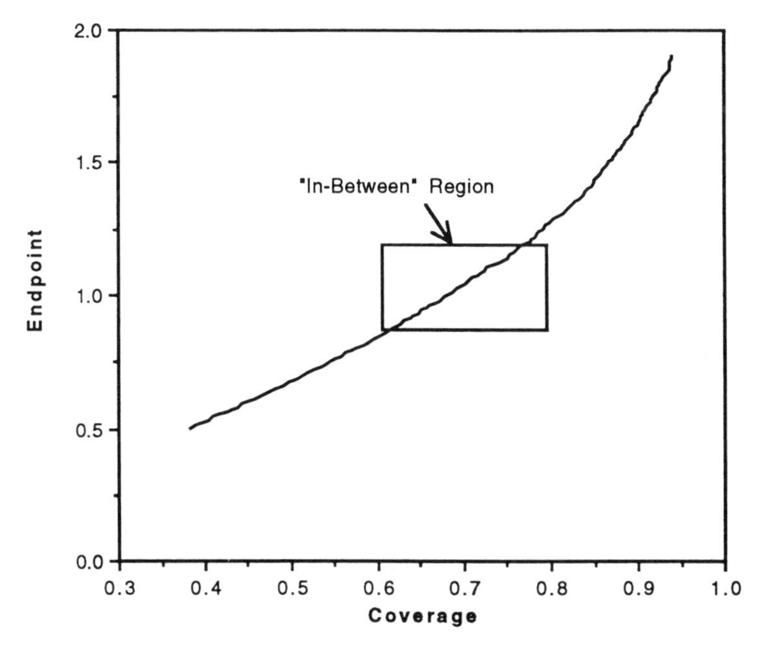

Figure 5.2. Endpoint of confidence intervals as a function of coverage.

50:50—50 percent coverage,
in between—75 percent coverage, and
very high—99 percent coverage.

This threefold division of uncertainty occurs in other fields. In American jurisprudence there are three levels of guilt.

"Probable cause"
"Clear and convincing evidence"
"Beyond a reasonable doubt"

A suspect can be bound over for trial if there is probable cause. In civil and many noncapital offenses, the standard is clear and convincing evidence. But, if the consequences of the decision are extremely drastic (like execution), the jury must find that guilt is proven beyond a reasonable doubt. (There is a fourth standard, "preponderance of evidence," but the difference between this and "clear and convincing" is not well established.)

There are situations in medical science where the use of a treatment that might be beneficial does not appear to have serious adverse reactions. In such a case, not much is lost by choosing a treatment that has a 50 percent chance of being effective. Most treatments (at least of outpatients) can be predicated on confidence intervals with coverage of 75 percent. Life-threatening events or procedures may need extreme evidence.

One minor thread needs to be addressed in this chapter. Proponents of the Neyman–Pearson formulation deride the current development in the medical literature that calls for confidence intervals instead of or in addition to hypothesis tests. They point out that confidence intervals are just another form of hypothesis tests. This belief is based on two things. The first is that the mathematical method used most often for computing the endpoints of a confidence interval is the same method as that used to compute a p-value. But just because two procedures use numerical integration does not mean that they are identical procedures. And that is all they have in common, a formal mathematical algorithm. Their scientific interpretation is much different.

The second reason proposed to show that hypothesis tests and confidence intervals are the same is based on a theorem by Erich Lehmann. Lehmann showed that if a uniformly most powerful test exists, then that test produces the shortest confidence interval for a given coverage. It is a neat theorem and its proof is one of those artistic gems of the mathematical literature that make reading the literature a pleasure. But it is an irrelevant finding. As Neyman pointed out, uniformly most powerful tests seldom exist, and they definitely do not exist in the setting of an RCT.

Chapters 6 to 11, which follow, develop the concept of restricted tests and show how they can be applied in the context of RCTs. Chapter 12 explores the use of Bayesian procedures to compute interval estimates of answers to medically defined questions. The final chapter uses data from a multiclinic study comparing two antidepressants to show how the sequence

restricted powerful hypothesis test,
medically defined questions, and
confidence interval answers

can be applied.

PART TWO

TECHNIQUES FOR APPLYING RESTRICTED TESTS TO DATA FROM RANDOMIZED CONTROLLED CLINICAL TRIALS

CHAPTER 6
Continuous Measures Taken over Time

6.1. An Example

Table 6.1 displays the results of exercise testing for 40 angina patients in a crossover study comparing drug A to placebo. Patients were given four exercise tests:

(1) week 0—just before randomization to treatment;
(2) week 4—at the end of the first double-blind period;
(3) week 5—at the end of a single-blind placebo wash-out; and
(4) week 9—at the end of the second double-blind period.

Half the patients were assigned placebo first, and half were assigned drug A first. Displayed are the seconds of exercise, under a standard protocol, until the patient was unable to continue due to angina pains.

Before examining the data more closely, we need an overall test of significance to determine whether there is a discernible "signal" in the midst of the random "noise." To construct this test of significance, we start with the null hypothesis:

H0: the probability distribution of time to end of exercise is independent of treatment.

This does not mean that the distribution of times is the same for each week. It could be that the distribution of times is different at week 9 from what it was at week 4. The null hypothesis only states that whatever differences there are in probability distribution, they are not affected by treatment.

Neyman has taught us that we also need a class of alternative hypotheses. To construct these, let us consider what is known about exercise testing

Table 6.1. Exercise Testing Times in a Two-Period Crossover

	Sequence group I: Week of study					Sequence group II: Week of study			
Patient number	0 SB Pcbo	4 Drug A	5 SB Pcbo	9 DB Pcbo	Patient number	0 SB Pcbo	4 DB Pcbo	5 SB Pcbo	9 Drug A
1	519	379	318	180	21	384	223	191	210
2	468	319	255	180	22	602	615	615	652
3	429	608	607	765	23	514	563	565	634
4	437	640	663	821	24	423	434	447	487
5	563	470	409	275	25	449	307	268	210
6	498	400	339	203	26	468	488	503	562
7	653	678	658	663	27	577	421	362	227
8	485	552	532	589	28	422	288	254	210
9	533	562	534	534	29	501	465	441	443
10	579	660	645	692	30	462	466	462	484
11	432	460	433	421	31	530	526	524	549
12	466	492	457	447	32	508	358	314	210
13	479	520	481	501	33	517	359	311	210
14	467	500	468	472	34	560	387	327	210
15	594	605	567	549	35	331	336	327	349
16	450	503	476	510	36	428	453	463	519
17	370	411	389	411	37	414	414	411	425
18	614	623	595	574	38	550	560	549	558
19	589	658	635	696	39	346	372	385	449
20	493	579	558	624	40	510	522	510	556

times in patients with angina. The most remarkable source of variability is what is often called the "training effect." That is, a patient's ability to exercise appears to change over time. In many cases, it improves (hence the name "training"). But, it does not always improve. It could deteriorate. Whichever occurs, it is clear that the rate at which these changes happen appears to be patient-specific.

So any reasonable alternative hypothesis has to take this into account. If we run a repeated-measures analysis of variance (ANOVA) on the data, then we are assuming that there is a consistent change across time that is the same for all patients. Thus, a repeated-measures ANOVA is inappropriate if we are seeking a powerful test. If we ignore the baselines (week 0 and week 5) and run a paired comparison of (drug A) − (placebo), we would confound a treatment difference with changes that occur across time. The fact that half the patients were randomized to drug A first means that a consistent pattern across time will tend to cancel out. However, because some patients might be improving and others deteriorating, this set of paired differences will include that variability in its variance, and our test statistic will lack power.

The fact that each patient is measured at three points in time, while on placebo, provides us with a means of estimating patient-specific patterns of change. With only three points, we cannot do much more than estimate a general linear trend across time, so the alternative hypothesis will have to be tuned to that rough an estimate. This leads us to an alternative hypothesis of the form:

H1: if $Y_i = A_i + B_i(t)$ represents the ith patient's trend across time (t), and if $Y_{di} = A_i + B_i(t_d)$, the expected value of Y_i at the end of treatment with drug A (at time t_d), and if X_d is the observed exercise time at t_d, then the expected value of X_{di} is greater than Y_{di}.

The null hypothesis is embedded in the class of alternatives by making

$$E(X_{di} - Y_{di}) = \Delta \text{ a single parameter of effect}$$

and noting that the null and alternative hypotheses become

$$\text{H0}: \Delta = 0$$

$$\text{H1}: \Delta > 0.$$

The significance test becomes a simple manipulation of the data

(1) Estimate A_i and B_i from the three placebo values for the ith patient.
(2) Predict the exercise testing time at the end of drug A treatment as Y_{di}, using A_i and B_i.
(3) Run a paired t-test on the differences $X_{di} - Y_{di}$.

The average difference from the data in Table 6.1 is 58.6 s, with a standard error of 13.02, yielding $t = 4.502$, significant evidence of a treatment effect. Furthermore, this analysis gives us some information to construct confidence intervals (CIs) about treatment effects:

$$50 \text{ percent CI on difference} = (49.8, 67.4),$$

$$75 \text{ percent CI on difference} = (43.6, 73.6),$$

$$99 \text{ percent CI on difference} = (25.0, 92.2).$$

Putting aside the question of whether exercise testing time has any real clinical relevance, these confidence intervals tell us that there is a 50:50 chance that the average improvement in a large population of similar patients will be 50 s or more, we can be reasonably sure that it will be 44 s or more, and we can be quite sure that it will not be as great as 100 s. Using this analysis, we can count how many patients had exercise times greater than predicted, or 20 percent greater than predicted. etc. We can identify a subset of "responders" and run a discriminant analysis to identify baseline characteristics that might predict "response." With this relatively precise measure of "response," we can find correlates among other measures.

Had we blindly analyzed the data in a repeated-measures ANOVA, the F-test for treatment would have been

$$F_{(1,38)} = 1.79, \quad p > 0.10$$

and we would have missed the evidence of efficacy that so obviously cries out from Table 6.1.

6.2. Restricted Tests Based on Observations over Time

6.2.1. General Methodology

What the preceding example shows is that a sequence of measurements taken over time on each patient provides a useful source of information upon which to construct a narrow class of reasonable alternative hypotheses. The one method of statistical analysis that seems particularly useless in this setting is the repeated-measures analysis of variance. To see why this is so, let us put the observations into a general mathematical setting: For the ith patient, we observe a sequence of values over time

$$X_{i1}, X_{i2}, X_{i3}, \ldots, X_{ik}.$$

This can be thought of as a vector or a k-dimensional random variable. If we assume that this random variable has a multidimensional Gaussian distribution, then the probability distribution is characterized by the vector of its means (k parameters) and the variance-covariance matrix ($k(k+1)/2$ parameters.) If we have to estimate these parameters from the data, we need considerably more than k^2 patients' data to allow for efficient estimation. Thus, if we observe each patient 12 times (once a week for a 12-week study), we need many more than 144 patients before we can even begin to estimate treatment differences. This is clearly not possible. If we cannot assume a Gaussian distribution, then we will have an even greater number of parameters to estimate.

We need, therefore, to find some way to reduce the complexity of the statistical models. The classical repeated-measures analysis of variance accomplishes this by assuming that the variance-covariance matrix is of a simple form that involves only two parameters. In this form, the variance across patients is the same at each measurement, all successive pairs have the same correlation, and measurements differing by more than one observation time are independent. The model also assumes that the mean vector is the same across all patients. These are difficult assumptions to justify in a clinical study.

In addition, the typical clinical study does not provide a neat complete vector of observations on all patients. The protocol may have called for patients to be seen once a week. But some patients miss a visit. Other patients come in after 10 days, or after 5 days, and the length of treatment varies by a week or more. It may not make sense to index these measurements by elapsed time but rather by cumulative dose of drug. It may not be possible to get some measurements at a given visit (and the reason for this may be pertinent to interpretation of treatment effects). Any method of analysis that requires that all patient records be forced into a straight-jacket of planned events will result in one of two arbitrary impositions. Either patients without complete "proper" records will be dropped from analysis, or patients with "improper" records will have their records modified so the computer program is fooled into thinking that they followed the protocol exactly.

Thus, we have a double problem in a clinical study. We need to reduce the description of the probability distribution of the vector of observations to one with a small number of parameters. And we need to have methods that allow us to use patients with "improper" patterns of observation. Recent theoretical work (see Laird, Lam, and Stam [1990]) has introduced what appears to be greater flexibility in the repeated-measures analysis of variance. The repeated values taken on a given patient are assumed to be representations of random variables that are independent of the random noise in the experiment but have been modified by a linear operator. So the model now consists of two parts,

an ordinary regression on independent measures, and
a linear regression on a set of random variables.

With this model, Laird and others have shown how to estimate the components of the model by means of maximum likelihood and how to derive statistical tests. However, for all its sophistication, the new expansion of repeated measures analysis of variance is still plagued by the need to assume that the vector of observations behaves consistently across all patients, and the subtle implications of assuming a linear operator for the random component force us to require unrealistic structures for the variance-covariance matrix.

Instead of forcing our data into an abstract mathematical model that is concocted with an eye toward having tractable mathematics, we should make use of biological models. Why do we follow patients across time anyway? Why not simply treat them for a period of time and take two measurements, one at baseline and one at final? We follow them over time because we expect the measurements to change over time and we hope to use those changes to characterize the dynamic relationship between treatment and patient. So before deciding how to analyze the data, it pays to give some thought to what we might expect to happen over time.

In Section 6.1, we looked at the use of a linear trend over time. Very often, this kind of a rough approximation of trend is adequate. If we have a sequence of observations over time, then a linear trend fitted to each patient's data provides us with

(1) a rough measure of overall change for each patient, and
(2) a means of using any patient with two or more observations.

In the example in Section 6.1, a linear trend was fit to a subset of the observations in order to take advantage of the crossover design. However, in a parallel study, where each patient is given a single treatment, the linear trend across all observations provides a measure of change that can be compared with two sample *t*-tests or one-way analyses of variance.

6.2.2. Acute Response over Time: Bronchodilator Example

It may be that there are enough observations to allow for a more sophisticated modeling of the effects of treatment over time. For instance, when a patient is given a single dose of a bronchodilator, we usually take spirometry measurements at selected points in time before dosing and thereafter at, say,

5 min post-dose,
15 min,
30 min,
60 min,
2 hrs,
3 hrs,
4 hrs, and
8 hrs.

Figure 6.1 shows plots of FEV-1 from individual patients given doses of a beta-agonist bronchodilator. It is obvious that there is no single overall pattern that can be found by averaging patient FEV-1s across each point in time. However, the sequence of times at which spirometry was taken

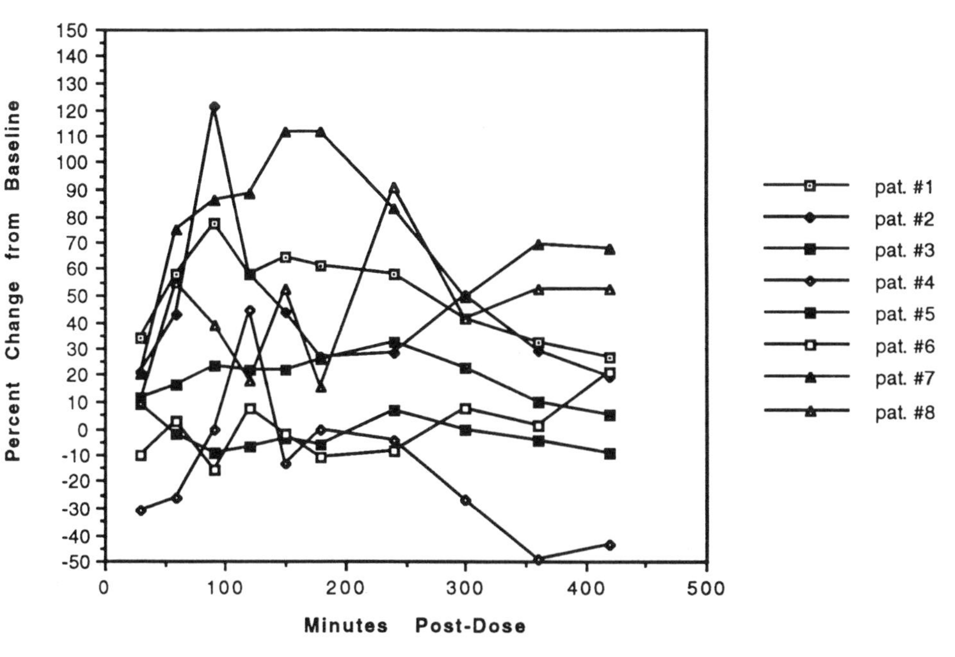

Figure 6.1. Percent change in FEV-1 following treatment.

was dictated by the expected pattern of pharmacological response. If the bronchodilator works, then we would expect to see an increase in FEV-1, peaking within the first hour and then dropping off over the next 7 hours. Why would one prefer a given bronchodilator to another one? One reason might be early onset of action. Another might be a longer duration of action. A third might be a greater level of activity. In Figure 6.2, we can sketch an ideal response pattern with these three aspects identified. Thus, it seems reasonable to derive four numbers from the time-course of observations for each patient:

(1) a time of onset of action,
(2) a measure of peak action,
(3) the duration of action, and
(4) overall "average" level of activity.

The essential idea here is that the expected way in which the treatment should act can be used to derive measures of "response" that are designed to detect that type of activity. In this example, a great deal needs to be done to adjust to vagaries in the data that will occur. A patient might suffer from acute bronchospasm during the trial and need relief medication, effectively stopping the sequence of FEV-1 measurements. So rules will be needed to enable the calculation of these three numbers from such a set of data. Since FEV-1 rises and falls spontaneously during the course of the day,

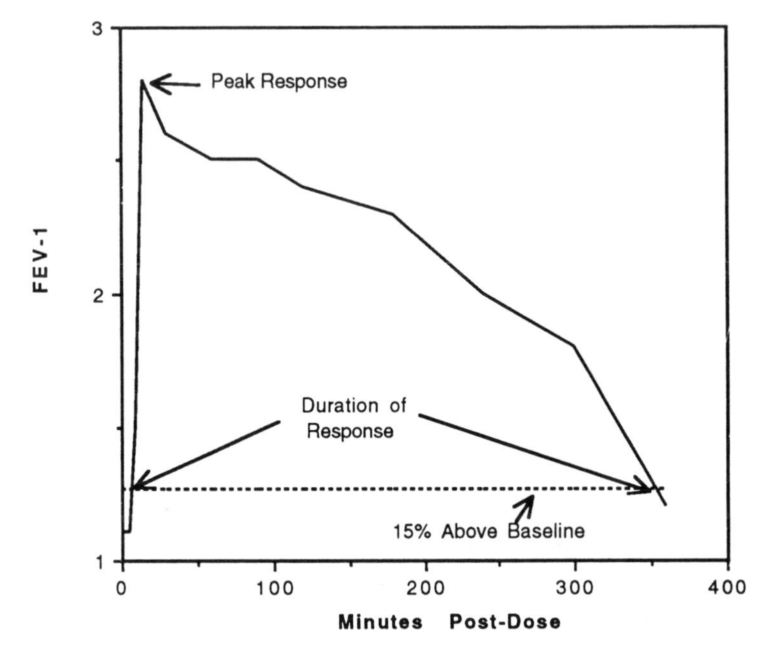

Figure 6.2. Ideal expected pattern of response to a single dose of a bronchodilator.

"onset" will have to be defined in terms of a clinically meaningful degree of change. "Duration" will also depend upon the end of this degree of change. Some patients are sure to have a response that continues to the end of the observations, so "duration" will need to be defined for such cases. But, all of these involve nothing more than a refinement of the basic medical/pharmacological expectation.

6.2.3. A Single Measure for Change over Time

Let us return to the problem of defining a single number as a "trend" over time. If we fit a straight line to each patient's data and use the slope of that line, it does not necessarily mean that we expect the response to be linear over time. If there is good reason to believe that response will not be linear over time, we might want to use some other value on the abscissa. For instance, if the dose of drug is titrated for each patient, we might want to use a weighted sum of the doses given up to time t in place of time t. Or if blood levels are available and the response is an immediate one, we might want to use blood levels. Thus, if there is enough known about the pharmacodynamics of the treatment, and if the right information has been collected, it might be possible to describe change in response as a linear function of change in some pharmacokinetic measure.

When the pharmacodynamics are not well characterized, we can use less specific knowledge about the expected response to generate a measure of change that is more sensitive to reasonable alternative hypotheses. Two examples are worth considering:

(a) Change is monotone over time.
(b) Observations are "disrupted" by wild and unusual events.

The observed measurements on a given patient can be thought of as the sum of two components

$$\text{Observation} = \text{Underlying trend} + \text{Random noise}.$$

Least squares linear slopes estimate the underlying trend and are the optimal procedure when the random noise has a symmetric and Gaussian distribution and the underlying trend is linear. However, this is seldom true. Very often the random noise is much more difficult to characterize, and it contains elements that influence the least squares estimator in an inappropriate way. There are several ways to use what is known about the expected response to improve on this.

It may be that the underlying trend may be monotone in one direction. A monotone nonincreasing function $g(t)$ is one such that if

$$t_1 < t_2$$

then

$$g(t_1) \geq g(t_2).$$

The observed values might look as in Figure 6.3. Brunk (Barlow, Bartholomew, Bremner, and Brunk [1972]) established an algorithm that finds the least squares estimator among the class of all monotone functions, and the Brunk estimator can be seen as a dotted line in Figure 6.3. The Brunk estimator can be used to estimate overall change by taking the final point on the estimated curve and subtracting the baseline from that or by fitting a straight line to the jump points of the Brunk estimator and taking its slope.

It may be that the overall response can be assumed to be monotone but that the random noise includes a few wild values due to events that are extraneous to the true nature of response. For instance, Figure 6.4 displays numbers of swollen and painful joints for a single patient in a 12-week study of rheumatoid arthritis. The week 4 value appears to be a flare that is out of line with the rest of the data. A trend line that is fit to the data will be strongly influenced by this single unusual value. The theory of robust estimation allows us to estimate the underlying trend line and to reduce the influence of outliers in the process. Figure 6.4 shows both the standard least squares line and a robust line. The slope of the robust line can be used as an indicator of change, which is more responsive to most of the data and less so to the unusual value at week 4.

Similarly, if the pharmacology or medical situation suggests it, we could

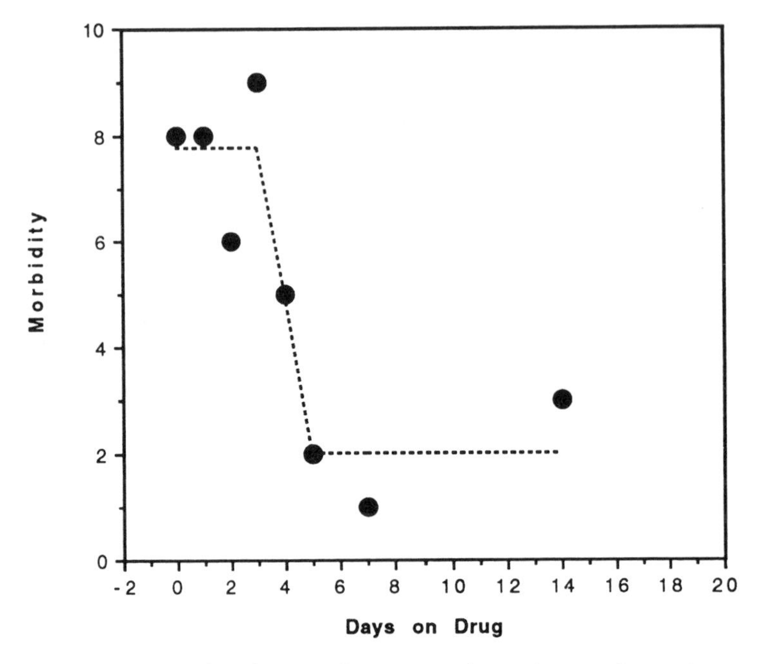

Figure 6.3. Brunk estimator of monotone decreasing trend over time.

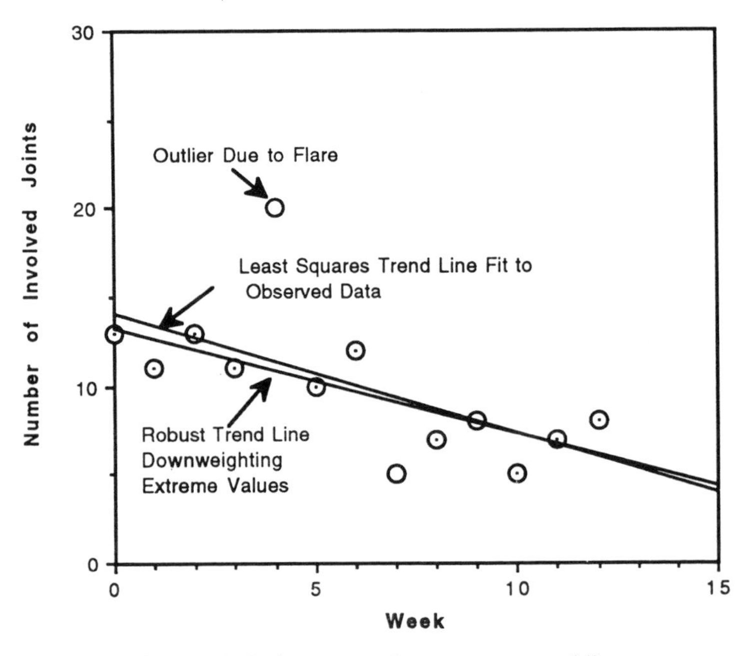

Figure 6.4. Robust versus least squares trend line.

fit individual patient data across time to other response patterns, like sigmoids, high-order polynomials, mixtures of exponentials, or shapes dependent upon theories of enzyme kinetics. The measures of change need not be overall slopes but can be time-associated with 50 percent change (similar to the ED-50 from animal pharmacology) or the average of the last three or four values from the best fitting estimated curve.

6.2.4. Summing Up

The important lesson to be learned is that we take observations over time because there is a good medical or scientific reason for looking at intermediate results. The existence of a scientific reason implies that, if the treatment works, it can be expected to produce a specific pattern or set of patterns of time-response. The average across time (the primary "treatment effect" in a repeated-measures ANOVA) or the differences (final-baseline) or the final value adjusted by analysis of covariance on the baseline are all measures that are conveniently produced by typical statistical programs on the computer. But they are seldom appropriate descriptors of what might be expected from an effective treatment. It usually makes for a more powerful significance test to first reduce each patient's record to a small set of patient-specific estimators of change that reflect what is expected.

CHAPTER 7

Combining Data Across Measures

7.1. An Example

Table 7.1 displays a sample of data from 10 patients treated for acute painful diabetic neuropathy. Ten patients were treated with placebo, and 10 were treated with an aldose-reductase inhibitor. At every clinic visit, each patient marked on 100-mm analog scales the maximum degree of discomfort felt during the previous week in terms of

(1) pain in the left foot,
(2) pain in the right foot,
(3) pain in the left calf,
(4) pain in the right calf,
(5) pain in the left thigh,
(6) pain in the right thigh,
(7) pain in the left hand,
(8) pain in the right hand,
(9) pain in the left arm,
(10) pain in the right arm,
(11)–(20) weakness in each of the above, and
(21)–(30) numbness in each of the above.

With a baseline and 6 clinic visits during the course of the study, this meant that 210 measures were collected for each patient on just this aspect of the disease. Table 7.1 displays the linear rates of change for the first 6 of these 30 measures (in the analysis of the full study, linear slopes were used to reduce the 210 measurements to 30 trends over time), along with two other trend lines. The first is the linear trend through the maximum value of each of the 30

Table 7.1. Least Squares Linear Rates of Change per Day Taken from Analog Distress Scores; Diabetic Neuropathy

Placebo-treated patients

Patient number	Self-rating of pain at sites: Foot		Calf		Thigh		Maximum distress	Dominant pain site
	Right	Left	Right	Left	Right	Left		
1	0.0095	0	−0.0023	0	−0.0543	0	−0.0461	−0.0543
2	−0.0041	−0.0042	0	0	−0.0083	−0.0002	−0.0058	−0.0042
3	0	0.0089	−0.0211	0.0035	0	0	−0.0565	−0.1429
4	−0.0553	−0.0303	0	0	0	0	−0.0698	−0.001
5	−0.0032	0.0057	0.0231	−0.0084	−0.0038	0.0043	−0.0047	0.0231
6	−0.0298	−0.0471	0	0	0	0	−0.0409	−0.0471
7	0.0233	0.0286	0.1227	0	0	0.0034	0.0689	0.0233
8	0.053	0.0137	−0.0043	0.0039	−0.0067	0	0.0658	0.0137
9	−0.0026	−0.0074	−0.0124	0.031	0	0	0.0168	0.031
10	0.0051	−0.0496	0.0024	0	0	0	−0.0522	−0.0667

Table 7.1 (*continued*)

Patient number	*Placebo-treated with drug B* Self-rating of pain at sites: Foot		Calf		Thigh		Maximum distress	Dominant pain site
	Right	Left	Right	Left	Right	Left		
11	−0.0056	−0.0758	0	0.0017	−0.0123	−0.0384	−0.0537	−0.0758
12	0	−0.0066	0	0	−0.0012	−0.0108	−0.0255	−0.0108
13	−0.012	−0.0991	−0.0082	−0.0045	−0.0689	−0.0665	−0.0197	−0.0991
14	0	−0.0547	0	0.0734	−0.2113	−0.0002	−0.1538	−0.2113
15	0	−0.011	−0.0021	−0.0051	−0.0077	−0.0077	0.0449	−0.0077
16	−0.02	−0.02	0	0	0	0	−0.02	−0.026
17	0.0026	0.0748	−0.0227	−0.1429	−0.0007	0.0043	0.6154	−0.1429
18	0	0	−0.0041	−0.0395	0	0.0003	−0.0395	−0.0395
19	−0.0318	−0.1458	0	0	−0.128	0.0004	−0.0817	−0.1458
20	−0.112	−0.0038	0	−0.0819	−0.0081	−0.0066	−0.005	−0.112

measurements at each visit. The second is the trend line through the symptom with the greatest baseline value (or the average of several if more than one had this greatest value). The first is labeled the "maximum distress" score. The second is labeled the "dominant symptom" score.

All 30 measures are comparable since they use the same basic measuring device. Later in this chapter, we will consider ways of standardizing measures that are in different scales in order to produce a combined score.

Diabetic neuropathy results in a mixed collection of symptoms that are all due to the same underlying pathology, the destruction of nerve tissue. As the nerves die away from the extremities, they send false messages, mostly of pain, but sometimes or more general dysathesias, including weakness and numbness. The classic medical picture is of successive deterioration from the distal to the proximal, and of vague general dysathesia, followed by pain, followed by numbness. However, not all patients follow this classic picture. The location and nature of these false messages vary from patient to patient and from time to time within a given patient. For this reason, it makes little sense to analyze the changes in a particular form of distress at a particular anatomical site. A comparison of treatments for changes in each of the 30 basic measures lacks power, since for any particular item, a large number of the patients show no distress at all during the study. What is needed is a measure of overall distress that combines each of the 30 measures and allows for this single measure to be applied to all patients.

An obvious single measure is the average of all 30 values. However, this is one case where the average is not very sensitive to treatment effects. Since the typical patient will not experience distress for more than half of these 30 symptoms/sites, the average will be very little influenced by those few types of distress that are giving the patient the most difficulty. The dominant symptom score recognizes this and picks that measure or those measures with the greatest distress at baseline. In this way, patients with pain in the left foot can be combined with patients whose greatest distress is due to weakness in the right leg, and so forth. The maximum distress score considers still another aspect of diabetic neuropathy. This is the fact that, for some patients, the exact nature of the distress changes from time to time. This is especially true for patients in early stages of the disease. One reason why diabetic neuropathy is often misdiagnosed early in its course is that the patient presents a vague collection of sometime symptoms (my big toe seems extra sensitive under the sheet at night, there is an intermittent burning pain in my thigh, my left foot feels like pins and needles, etc.). The maximum for each of the rating scales represents an outer envelope of illness severity. The exact symptom that forms the maximum will differ from patient to patient and may differ from week to week with the same patient, but it is a medically reasonable measure of neuropathy.

Two-sample *t*-tests comparing the dominant symptom least squares (L.S.) rates of change and the maximum distress L.S. rates of change both show

Table 7.2. Two-Sample T-Tests Based on Data in Table 7.1

Measure of effect	Average slopes: Placebo	Average slopes: Drug B	Pooled variance	t-test	Significance
Pain in right foot	−0.00041	−0.0204	0.00083	1.554	0.079
Pain in left foot	−0.00817	−0.03508	0.00174	0.25	0.404
Pain in right calf	0.01329	−0.00371	0.00161	0.949	0.185
Pain in left calf	0.00152	0.02481	0.00124	1.674	0.066
Pain in right thigh	−0.00731	−0.02982	0.0024	1.027	0.167
Pain in left thigh	0.00075	−0.00135	0.00222	0.099	0.462
Maximum distress	−0.01245	−0.10144	0.00246	4.008	0.002
Dominant pain site	−0.02251	−0.08709	0.00302	2.626	0.015

Table 7.3. Confidence Intervals on Percent Reduction in Maximum Distress and Dominant Pain Site: Drug B versus Placebo

Measure	Average percent change after 6 weeks, treatment: Placebo	Average percent change after 6 weeks, treatment: Drug B
Maximum distress	−5.23	−42.61
Dominant pain site	−9.45	−36.58

Difference in effect of drug B versus placebo

Measure	Lower confidence bounds 99%	Lower confidence bounds 75%	Lower confidence bounds 50%	Median difference	Upper confidence bounds 50%	Upper confidence bounds 75%	Upper confidence bounds 99%
Maximum distress	6.12	25.54	30.8	37.38	43.75	49.21	68.63
Dominant pain site	−7.51	14.02	19.84	27.12	34.41	40.23	61.76

significant differences between treatments. But none of the comparisons for individual symptoms show such a result. See Table 7.2. Having established that there is a significant difference between treatments, we can go on to Table 7.3, which displays 50 percent, 75 percent and 99 percent confidence intervals for the mean differences in the percent improvement at the end of the study, projected from the mean slopes and mean baselines,

$$\% \text{ improvement} = 100 \text{ (slope/week) (6 weeks)/(baseline)},$$

for both dominant symptom and maximum distress.

7.2. Reducing Many Measures to a Few

7.2.1. General Methodology

Although the current methods of statistical analysis usually focus on a single or small group of efficacy parameters, a randomized clinical trial is really an exercise in which we accumulate a great deal of information on each patient at each visit. An appropriate statistical analysis of these data should make use of all or almost all of that information. We collect these data because we think that they bear upon the medical questions that will be examined in the study, and we have an obligation to examine them in order to see how they can be used to answer specific medical questions.

The basic principle of analysis proposed in this book is that we first create a small number (hopefully only one) of powerful significance tests that can determine whether there is enough information in the data to distinguish between treatments. Once significance is found, the individual elements of data can be examined more carefully, using the tools of confidence intervals to describe what it was that differed between the treatments. One way to do this might be to pick the "most important" of the efficacy parameters and run the significance tests on those. This is reflected in the tendency to identify the "primary" efficacy variables in the protocol of the randomized controlled trial.

In some cases, this is a reasonable procedure. When comparing antihypertensive medications, the "primary" efficacy variable is often the change in systolic or diastolic blood pressure. However, for many chronic diseases, the disease is best described as a syndrome of signs and symptoms, and beneficial change may be reflected in some combination of these signs and symptoms. It may not be clear what that combination might be at the time the study is designed. Often, a large clinical study in some chronic disease is not only the first time a new treatment is being compared but also the first time a large number of patients are followed under careful supervision for a reasonable period of time. So the RCT that compares two treatments may also be the best source available for characterizing the time-course of the disease. In such a case, the paradigm that divides studies into "exploratory" and "confirmatory" studies makes no sense. The one large study will have to be used to define reasonable summary measures of efficacy and, at the same time, use those measures to test whether there is a difference between treatments.

This is, in fact, what Fisher did in his agricultural papers (see Fisher [1921,1926] for examples). Such (now standard) methods as regression analysis, ANOVA, ANCOVA, and orthogonal polynomials first appear as methods of analysis derived to fit the data that accumulated in specific trials. The overall significance test that emerges from such "data dredging" might be influenced by random glitches in the data, so the analyst has to carefully balance between doing what appears to make biological sense and following what may very well be nothing more than Anscombe's [1985] Will o' the Wisps. A later chapter of this book deals with a method for maintaining a reasonably correct p-value to the significance test, while still deriving the summary measure(s) from the data. For the moment, then, let us assume that the summary measure(s) can be developed independently of the data in the study to be analyzed.

In general, there are two ways of developing a useful summary measure. We can use the techniques of multivariate statistics to examine the entire vector of observations as a point in some large dimensional space. Or we can combine across elements of the vector to find a medically meaningful summary measure(s) of one dimension. Postponing multivariate methods, let us consider methods for summarizing across measures.

What are some useful and medically reasonable summary measures?

7.2.2. Combining Measures in the Same Scale

The example (in Section 7.1) showed how several measures on the same scale can be combined by considering the maximum distress at each visit or by following the dominant baseline symptom. Deriving a measure under such circumstances should depend on why the several measures were taken simultaneously. If they were taken because the disease being examined has a number of similar symptoms that may or may not occur in a given patient, then it might be best to derive a combination of the more extreme values, as in the example. On the other hand, the several measures may represent different aspects of the same general biological function and all might be expected to reflect on the state of the disease for every patient, so a linear combination will be best.

For instance, studies of antihypertensives traditionally take both systolic and diastolic pressures in at least two positions (standing and supine.) This is done because different types of medication work on different parts of the cardiovascular system, and the relative relationships across these four measures are expected to characterize the patients' response. In some cases, the type of medication can be expected to work best on one particular measure (alpha blockers on standing diastolic), so the measure most sensitive to the expected activity of treatment can be chosen directly. In other cases, the treatment can be expected to modify the normal relationship between systolic and diastolic or between supine and standing pressures, so some contrast or correlation analysis may, in fact, be the one most sensitive to detecting treatment differences.

Another example occurs with acute response to a bronchodilator. The spirometer creates a graph of flow rate versus volume or expiration versus time (see Figure 7.1). From this graph, we pick off a set of measures like

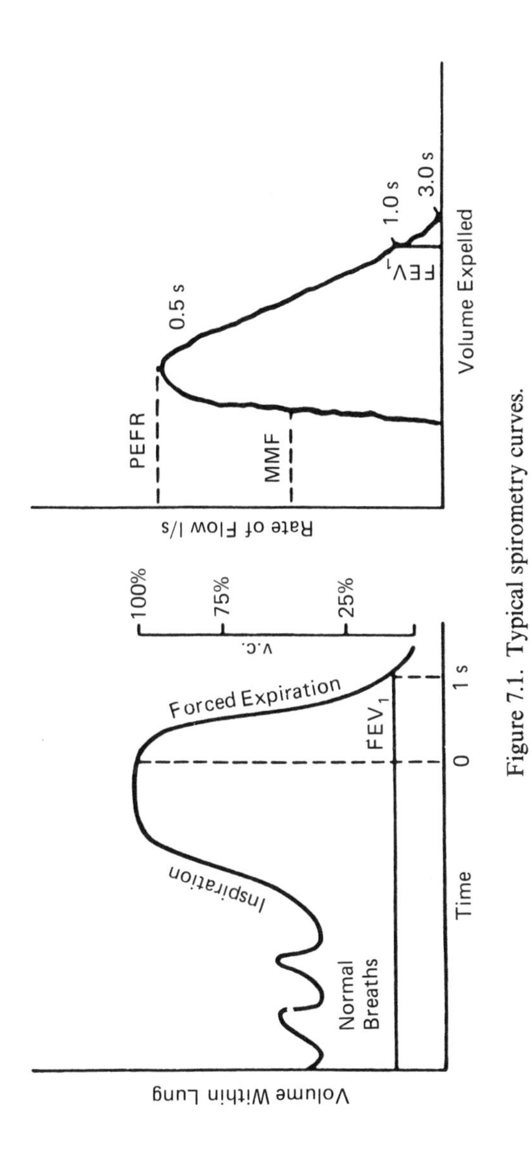

Figure 7.1. Typical spirometry curves.

FEV-1, FEV-3, FVC, MEFR, FEFxx-yy, etc. The volume measures are all in the same scale (liters), and the rate measures are all in the same scale (liters per minute). Each of these measures was developed as a diagnostic tool, but when they are used to track the effects of treatment, the differences in meaning associated with specific diagnoses may not be important. In a survey of placebo effects from several studies (Salsburg [1981]), it was shown that changes in all these measures are highly correlated, so any one of them contains as much information as all the others (at least with respect to changes in a patient's condition). The "best" measure is, then, the one that is most sensitive to the expected treatment effect and has a small variance within-patient. In the data examined, this turned out to be the FVC (a measure that is usually considered medically to be relatively useless for diagnosis).

Thus, the choice of summary measures from a set of measurements in the same scale involves an interplay between the expected effects of the treatment, what is known about changes in the disease, and the statistical properties of the change scores of the individual measurements.

7.2.3. Combining Measures with Different Scales

Although the previous cases described situations where several measurements are all on the same scale, it is more usual to have a set of measurements that are on different scales (nerve conductance velocities in m/s, sensory maps in cm, global ratings on a four-point scale, etc.). How these can be combined into a single summary measure depends upon whether their combination has some medical or pharmacological meaning. As with more homogeneous measures, it may be best to choose a small number of them to be used as primary measures by themselves. However, if all are equally important (or all equally lacking in clear-cut medical value), then it is possible to put them all on the same scale and combine them.

One way to make different measures comparable is to standardize them to dimensionless measures of the form

$$Y = (X\text{-standard})/\text{scale}.$$

The standardized normal variate

$$Y = (X\text{-mean})/\text{S.D.}$$

is the prototype of this. But the standardization need not be done with averages and standard deviations. All we need is to establish a value, "standard," about which the measure can be expected to vary, and another value, "scale," that divides out the units of measure and that keeps all the standardized variables within the same range of values. For instance, if

$$F = \text{final value taken after treatment,}$$

$$B = \text{baseline value taken before treatment}$$

then

$$Y = 100(F - B)/B$$

is a standardized variate that is easily seen to be the percent change from baseline. When spirometry measures are "corrected" for predicted, the result is a percent of predicted and is standardized. So the idea of standardizing measurements that are originally on different scales is widely used in medicine. Another method involves picking two ideal values, A and B, between which a measurement should range in a healthy person. Then

$$Y = (X - A)/(B - A), \quad \text{where } X = \text{the original measurement}$$

is a standardized measure of the deviation beyond this normal range.

Once a set of measurements has been standardized, they can be combined as described in the previous section for measurements with a common scale.

An alternative approach (which is a form of standardization based on relative ordering) was proposed by O'Brien [1984]. We order each of the measurements across all patients (who have that measurement) and replace the observed value, Xi for the ith patient, with the relative rank

$$Ri = \text{Rank}(Xi)/N, \quad N = \text{number of patients with that measurement.}$$

The use of a possibly variable N allows us to provide a relative rank score for each observed variable for each patient. For instance, suppose we have collected patient self-ratings of pain along with analgesic usage. However, some patients failed to bring back their bottles of escape analgesic, so while we may have self-ratings of pain on all patients, we have analgesic usage on only 75 percent of them. If there are 100 patients in the study (across all treatment groups), the relative rank for self-rating of pain uses a divisor of 100 and the relative rank for analgesic usage uses a divisor of 75.

O'Brien then proposed that each patient have a summary measure, which is the average of all the relative ranks for that patient. Since the rankings were done across all treatment groups, this summary measure can be used to compare treatments. However, we do not need to stop with the average of the relative ranks. Hajek [1968] proposed a set of test statistics for the comparison of treatments where the relative rank is converted to a score by taking a function of that rank

$$Y_i = f(R_i), \quad \text{for some smooth function } f(\ ).$$

For instance,

$$Y_i = R_i^4,$$

$$Y_i = \log(R_i),$$

$$Y_i = 0 \text{ if } R_i < 0.8,\ 1 \text{ if } R_i \geq 0.8.$$

The first and third (Conover and Salsburg [1988]) of these are the optimum scores for detecting a difference where the treatment affects only a subset of the patients. The second one is the Savage score (Conover [1980]) and is the optimum score for detecting a treatment effect in the form of a Lehmann shift.

A Lehmann shift would occur if the measurement has a natural upper bound and the treatment tends to drive the patient toward that bound. For instance, in exercise testing for angina patients, there is a natural upper bound in the sense that a patient restored to perfect health may not be able to exercise beyond 600 s. So it becomes more and more difficult to produce a treatment effect, the higher the patient's baseline. If we expect the treatment to improve a patient's exercise time better than he will improve on placebo, Savage scores may be the most powerful procedure.

On the other hand, if we expect only a subset of patients to respond to treatment for any single measurement, then an average of either of the other scores will be a powerful single summary measure.

The third score described here would be less powerful than the first, in general, because it reduces a continuous variable to a discrete one. However, it has the advantage of being easily interpreted. If we standardize the ranks and run this score, it means that each patient's score is the percent of measurements for which that patient's change is in the upper 80th percentile. In some general sense, we can think of this as a definition of "response," and the score becomes the percent of measurements on which the patient responds.

This brings us to a final summary statistic that tends to be quite powerful and is easily interpreted medically. For each measurement, establish a clinically meaningful change. For instance, we might require that a patient's systolic blood pressure drop by 10 mm Hg or more before it is considered "clinically meaningful." Then convert each measure to a (0, 1) score of the form

$$Y_i = \begin{cases} 1 & \text{if } X_i \geq \text{a clinically meaningful change,} \\ 0 & \text{otherwise.} \end{cases}$$

The average value of the Y_is for a given patient is the percentage of measures on which that patient had a clinically meaningful change.

7.3. Treating Many Measures as a Vector

7.3.1. General Principles

Suppose we have some means of measuring five symptoms on a CHF patient: ankle edema, dyspnea, fatigue, 50-feet walking time, and ejection fraction. We can view these five separate measures as a single thing, a vector, symbolized as

$$\mathbf{x} = \begin{bmatrix} x^1 \\ x^2 \\ x^3 \\ x^4 \\ x^5 \end{bmatrix} = \begin{bmatrix} \text{aedema} \\ \text{dyspnea} \\ \text{fatigue} \\ \text{50-feet walk time} \\ \text{ejection frac.} \end{bmatrix}.$$

It is convenient to think of this vector as a point in five-dimensional space. No one is able to visualize five dimensions, but it is adequate for purposes of analogy to visualize it as a point in three dimensions. In this way, a set of patients' vectors can be visualized as a cluster of points. If two groups of patients differ, we can think of them as two clusters of points (with perhaps some overlap.)

To understand the geometry of vectors, we construct three-dimensional pictures, where a high dimensional vector is depicted as a directed line with an arrowhead and spaces of lower dimension are depicted as planes. As you construct these three-dimensional analogs, it rapidly becomes clear that you cannot extend many of the ideas associated with one-dimensional numbers. The points in a vector space do not have a natural ordering. Distances are directional, and three points that are equidistant from each other can be in an infinite number of configurations. Other concepts from one-dimensional statistics also undergo mutations.

For instance, the average of a set of one-dimensional numbers can be extended to the average of a set of points. This is done by averaging all the values associated with each component of the vector. In the example, the average for the CHF patients described earlier is a point whose first dimension is the average ankle edema score, whose second dimension is the average dyspnea score, etc. Analogous to the standard deviation of a set of numbers is the variance-covariance matrix of a set of vectors. The variance-covariance matrix is a square array of numbers, calculated by taking pairwise products of the components of the vectors. Less important than how it is calculated is to recognize that what was once a single number (standard deviation) is now replaced by a square array of numbers.

7.3.2. The Multivariate Normal Distribution

The analogy to one-dimensional numbers that holds up best is the multivariate normal distribution. The one-dimensional normal distribution is one of those neat mathematical constructions whose beauty and attraction lie in the interrelationships of its elements. It is the limit of the central limit theorem. Sums of normally distributed variables have a normal distribution. The average and sample variance of a set of normally distributed numbers are statistically independent. Among all possible distributions, the normal is the only one that has a number of simple linear-type properties.

The multidimensional analog of the univariate normal distribution is one of the great and beautiful creations of mathematical statistics. Its parameters are the mean vector and the variance-covariance matrix. It is the only multivariate distribution all of whose subdistributions belong in the same family and all of whose conditional distributions belong in the same family. There is a multivariate central limit theorem, and the multivariate normal is its limit. There are multivariate analogs of the standard normal theory methods. Analogous to the t-test is Hotelling's T^2. Multivariate analysis of variance (MANOVA) is derived from a simple generalization of analysis of variance. Analogous to the chi-square distribution (sums of squares of normal variates) is the Wishart distribution. The list goes on. The multivariate normal has captivated the imaginations of some of this century's best mathematical minds. Great textbooks have been written on the subject. In 1988, over 200 articles dealing with the multivariate normal distribution appeared in the journals covered by the *Current Index to Statistics.*

Unfortunately, significance tests based on the multivariate normal distribution are of little use in clinical research.

There are two reasons for this. The first is that, with one exception, all the multivariate normal significance tests are sensitive to departures from normality. As in the univariate case, this usually means that the test lacks power to detect fairly obvious differences between treatment groups, if the underlying distributions are not normal. For instance, suppose one treatment group produces points tightly clustered together (in our three-dimensional visualization) and the other produces points that gather in a large half-shell outside of but around part of this cluster. (See Figure 7.2 for a two-dimensional view of this.) The multivariate normal distribution implies that all points would cluster in symmetric ellipsoids, so such a situation cannot arise in a normal distribution. A normal theory test would first act as if the two clusters of points came from the same shaped ellipsoid, filling in the "missing" part of the ellipsoid for the second set of points in and among the cluster from the first set. Then it would compare the average positions of the two ellipsoids and find them almost on top of one another.

Most of the data collected in clinical studies are bounded, skewed, discrete, or have regions of impossible values. All of these characteristics preclude the multivariate normal. So we know from medical and pharmacological considerations that these data will not be normally distributed.

There is one exception to this sensitivity of multivariate normal tests to nonnormality. Efron [1969] has shown that the one-sample Hotelling's T^2 test is robust against many nonnormal distributions. Thus, if we have a set of vectors from a single treatment group or if we run a crossover study and collect complete vectors at each treatment on each patient, we can use the difference between treatments as a single vector. If we have such a situation, we can test the null hypothesis that the mean vector has some preset value (such as all zeros).

But the second problem with multivariate normal significance tests is

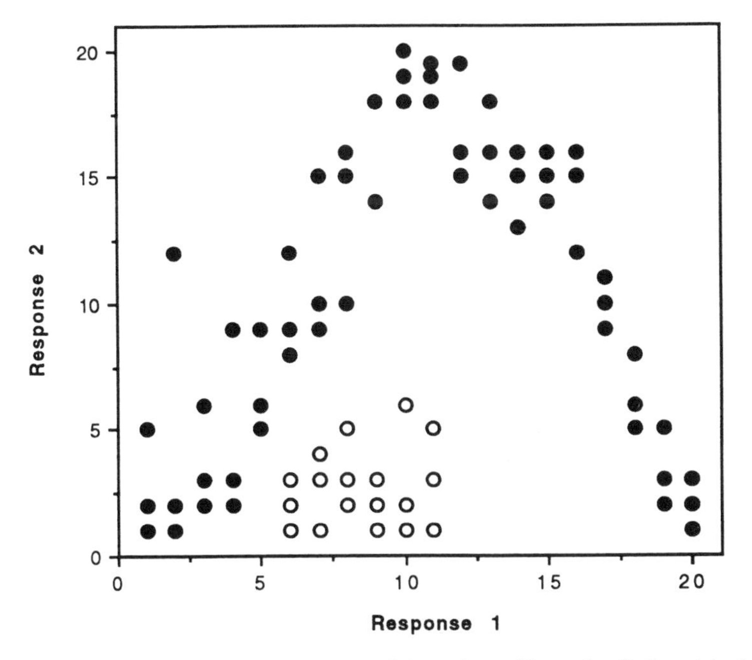

Figure 7.2. Example of two separate sets of data that will not be distinguished with multivariate normal theory tests.

that it is difficult, if not impossible, to construct restricted versions of those tests. All the standard multivariate normal tests compare the observed mean vectors to single preset vectors or to each other and are equally powerful against all possible deviations in any direction in any dimension. This is even true for the one-sample Hotelling's T^2. Attempts have been made (Chinchilli and Sen [1981]) to derive restricted versions of some of these tests, but they are quite difficult to translate into medically sensible hypotheses.

7.3.3. Nonparametric Multivariate Methods

Most one-dimensional nonparametric procedures start by ordering the observations and then comparing the ranks of observations among treatments. There is no unique way of ordering all the points in a multidimensional space. So methods of nonparametric analysis have had to settle for partial orderings, often based on arbitrary characteristics.

If we think of the vectors as points in multidimensional space (but visualize them as points in three dimensions), we can consider each point as the center of a series of concentric spheres, with increasing radii. These sphere define "neighbors."

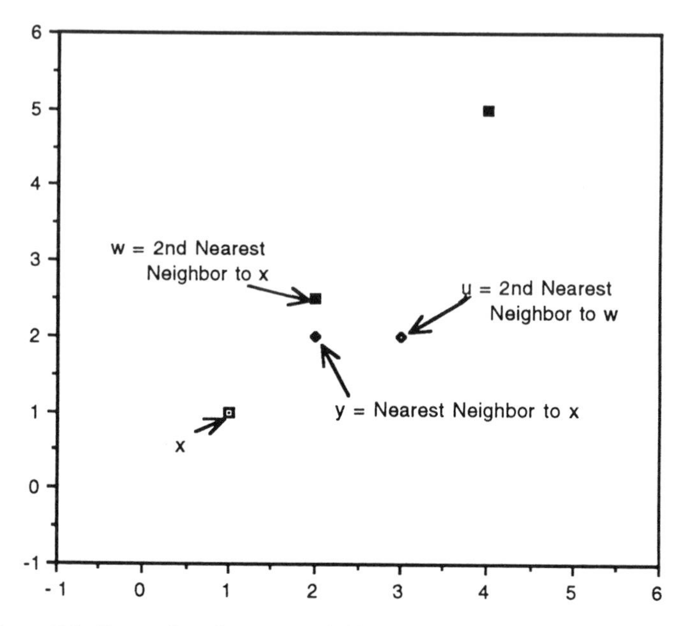

Figure 7.3. Examples of nearest neighbors and second nearest neighbors.

7.3.3.1. Nearest Neighbor Tests

Fixing the radii of the spheres requires that we impose preconceived distances on the data. This means that our test may be sensitive to arbitrary decisions about scaling (for instance, we might get different results if we measure walking time in seconds than if we measure it in minutes). To avoid this problem, we can consider the concept of "nearest neighbors" (Henze [1988]). The nearest neighbor to a given point, **x**, is that point, **y**, whose distance to **x** is less than or equal to the distance from any other point to **x**. It is possible for **y** to be the nearest neighbor of several points. In the example displayed in Figure 7.3, **y** is the nearest neighbor to **x** and to **w**. The second nearest neighbor to **x** is another point, **w**, such that there is only one other point that **w** is closer to than it is to **x**. Again, **y** can be the second nearest neighbor to several points. In general, the kth nearest neighbor to a point **x** is a point **v** such that there are exactly $k - 1$ other points that are nearer to **x** than **v** is.

This seems like a complicated way of ordering data, but it has an advantage over many other methods. If we have two sets of points (placebo versus drug A), under the null hypothesis that the two sets of points have the same probability distribution, the number of points from the same set that are kth nearest neighbors to each other has an easily derived probability distribution. This is the multivariate nearest neighbor significance test of Henze. It is powerful against an alternative where at least one of the two treatment groups produces points in a tight cluster.

What makes this type of test useful in clinical studies is that effective treatment often forces many measures of disease to "march along" together. That is, patients on an effective drug often respond in a stereotypical fashion, while those on placebo tend to produce a scatter of improvements on some measures and not on others. The vectors of change in these measurements will, then, tend to cluster tightly together for the treated group and to be more loosely scattered for the placebo group.

7.3.3.2. Projection Tests

Another method of deriving nonparametric tests is to find some way to string the points out along a one-dimensional line. One method uses the minimum spanning tree (Friedman and Rafsky [1983]). Again, we visualize the two sets of points in space (one set from each treatment group). We can connect the points so that there is a line segment between any two points. This is called a spanning tree if all points are connected and if only one line connects any two points (see Figure 7.4). The size of the spanning tree is the sum of the lengths of the line segments connecting the points. For any finite set of points, there is a unique spanning tree of minimum size, the minimum spanning tree.

If the minimum spanning tree were a single broken line, we could order the points along the tree from one end to the other. But, in most cases,

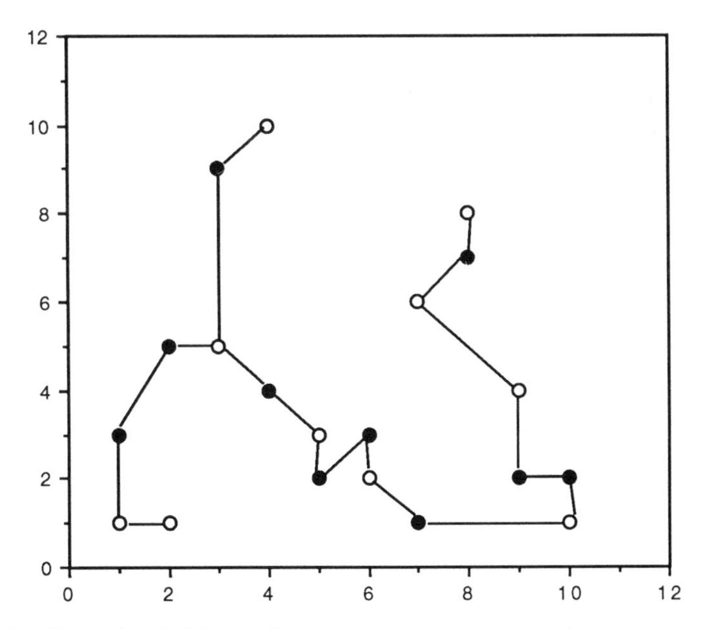

Figure 7.4. Example of minimum distance spanning tree connecting two sets of points.

there are branches leading out from the main tree, and it is sometimes difficult to identify the "main tree." Friedman and Rafsky have derived a set of rules for ordering the points along such a tree in an arbitrary fashion. Once such an ordering is created, then we can treat the order as univariate ranks and run the standard nonparametric rank tests.

A problem with the Friedman-Rafsky approach is that the ordering of the points is a fortuitous result of the way the data fall. It is not clear what the ordering is powerful against. If we use it to do a runs test, then it is powerful against the situation where at least one of the two groups is tightly clustered (as in the Henze nearest neighbor test). But the Wilcoxon test on this ordering will be powerful only if the two sets of points tend to be in separate clusters.

However, the idea of ordering the points with respect to a line in space can be used to construct a well-defined directed test. Again, visualize the points in space (see Figure 7.5). There is some region of space that is "bad" in the sense that a patient whose vector lies there has deteriorated. There is also some region that is "good." If these regions can be identified, then we can go further and identify a single "bad" point and a single "good" point and connect the two with a line. Any other point in space can be projected down onto this line. Its image is the point on the line nearest to it. The points can now be ordered by their projections and the usual nonparametric rank tests run on their projections.

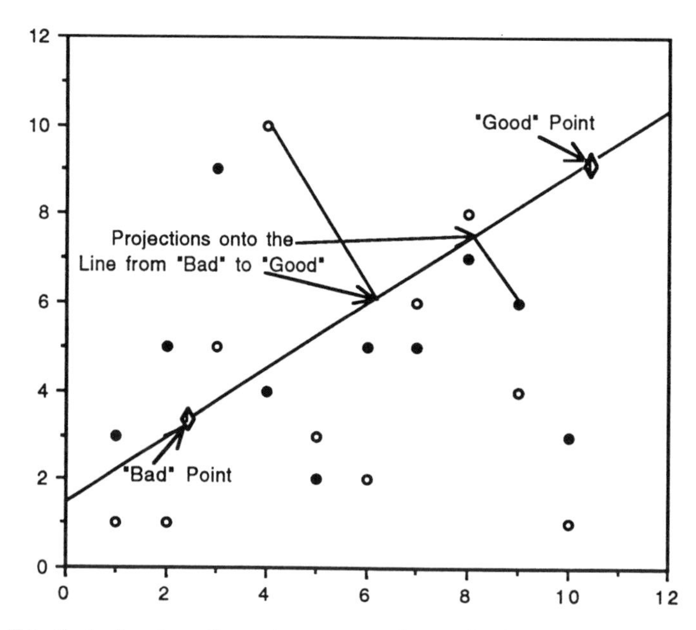

Figure 7.5. Reducing two dimensions to one by projections onto a line defined in terms of expected clinical response.

But a projection of a point onto a line is nothing but a linear combination of the components of that vector. Thus, our test score, derived in this geometric analogy, is, in fact, a weighted sum of the individual measures. This brings us back to the techniques discussed in Section 7.2. However, this use of a geometric analogy can help develop a medically meaningful score or weighted sum. Rather than dreaming up arbitrary weights to create a possibly useful index, the geometry can be used to visualize the points associated with a prototypical deteriorating patient and a prototypical improving patient. The geometry then automatically creates the correct weighting scheme.

Projection tests are designed to make use of the expected medical or pharmacological response to treatment, and they are best used where the medical scientists designing the RCT can agree on a reasonable pattern of expected response. Remember, the basic idea behind the use of restricted test is that we can describe a small class of alternative hypotheses (what is expected to happen if there is a treatment difference). If the designers of the RCT cannot agree on a general pattern of expected "response," then it is sometimes useful to draw up a group of patient scenarios, describing possible outcomes for specific patients (perhaps even using historical data to produce the patterns of "response" from actual patients). Then the designers can divide these scenarios into three categories

(1) those representing "response,"
(2) those representing "no response," and
(3) others.

The average vector of observations from the first group can be used as the "good" point, and the average vector of observations from the second group can be used as the "bad" point.

CHAPTER 8
Counts of Events

8.1. An Example

Table 8.1 displays data from 200 "patients" that were generated from a random model on the computer. The patients are divided into 10 "clinics" with 20 patients each. They are also subdivided into four "severity" classes at baseline. Finally, they are divided into "smokers" and "nonsmokers." Table 8.1 displays the total numbers of patients in each category of

$$(\text{Clinic}) \times (\text{Severity Class}) \times (\text{Smoking Status}) \times (\text{Treatment})$$

along with the numbers of patients with "events" in those categories.

This computer-generated "study" can be thought of as mimicking a clinical study of patients with angina who were treated with placebo or test drug and followed for a period of time. The "event" can be thought of as the occurrence of some specific cardiovascular morbidity.

To generate these numbers, each "patient" had a 30 percent chance of being in class 1, 40 percent in class 2, 20 percent in class 3, and 10 percent in class 4. There was a 40 percent chance that the patient would be a "smoker." Nonsmokers on placebo had the following probabilities of event, depending upon baseline severity class:

Class	Probability
1	0.20
2	0.25
3	0.35
4	0.45

Nonsmokers in the treated group had the following probabilities of event,

Table 8.1. Counts of Patients with Events

Clinic	Severity classes	Smoke	Placebo X	Placebo N	Treatment X	Treatment N	Clinic	Severity classes	Smoke	Placebo X	Placebo N	Treatment X	Treatment N
1	1	Yes	1	2	0	3	6	1	Yes	0	1	0	2
1	1	No	0	0	1	1	6	1	No	0	0	0	2
1	2	Yes	3	6	2	4	6	2	Yes	0	1	0	1
1	2	No	0	0	1	1	6	2	No	1	1	1	1
1	3	Yes	0	2	0	1	6	3	Yes	1	2	0	1
1	3	No	0	0	0	0	6	3	No	0	1	0	0
1	4	Yes	0	0	0	0	6	4	Yes	3	3	0	0
1	4	No	0	0	0	0	6	4	No	0	1	1	3
2	1	Yes	1	2	1	1	7	1	Yes	0	2	0	1
2	1	No	0	0	1	4	7	1	No	0	0	0	0
2	2	Yes	1	7	0	1	7	2	Yes	2	3	1	4
2	2	No	0	0	0	2	7	2	No	0	1	2	3
2	3	Yes	0	0	0	1	7	3	Yes	0	2	0	0
2	3	No	0	0	0	1	7	3	No	1	1	0	1
2	4	Yes	1	1	1	1	7	4	Yes	1	1	1	1
2	4	No	0	0	0	0	7	4	No	0	0	0	0
3	1	Yes	2	4	0	0	8	1	Yes	0	3	0	0
3	1	No	0	1	0	0	8	1	No	0	0	0	0
3	2	Yes	1	2	0	3	8	2	Yes	0	4	1	5
3	2	No	0	0	0	0	8	2	No	1	2	1	1
3	3	Yes	0	1	0	1	8	3	Yes	0	1	0	1
3	3	No	1	1	0	4	8	3	No	0	0	1	1
3	4	Yes	1	1	0	0	8	4	Yes	0	0	0	1
3	4	No	0	0	1	1	8	4	No	0	0	1	1
4	1	Yes	0	1	0	1	9	1	Yes	1	3	0	0

Table 8.1 (*continued*)

Clinic	Severity classes	Smoke	Placebo		Treatment		Clinic	Severity classes	Smoke	Placebo		Treatment	
			X	N	X	N				X	N	X	N
4	1	No	0	0	0	0	9	1	No	2	3	0	0
4	2	Yes	1	4	0	3	9	2	Yes	0	2	1	3
4	2	No	0	1	2	3	9	2	No	2	2	0	1
4	3	Yes	0	0	0	2	9	3	Yes	0	0	0	1
4	3	No	2	2	0	0	9	3	No	0	0	1	2
4	4	Yes	0	1	1	1	9	4	Yes	0	0	1	3
4	4	No	1	1	0	0	9	4	No	0	0	0	0
5	1	Yes	0	1	0	0	10	1	Yes	0	2	0	0
5	1	No	1	2	0	0	10	1	No	1	4	0	0
5	2	Yes	0	2	1	5	10	2	Yes	2	4	0	1
5	2	No	1	2	0	2	10	2	No	0	0	0	1
5	3	Yes	0	1	0	1	10	3	Yes	0	0	0	1
5	3	No	1	1	0	0	10	3	No	0	0	0	0
5	4	Yes	0	1	0	1	10	4	Yes	0	0	2	7
5	4	No	0	0	0	1	10	4	No	0	0	0	0

depending upon baseline severity class:

Class	Probability
1	0.10
2	0.10
3	0.10
4	0.25

If a patient was a "smoker," the probability of event increased by 0.30, across the board. If we were to ignore the classifications of patients (by baseline severity and smoking status), these probabilities were chosen so that a simple Fisher's exact test comparing the overall incidence of events between treatment groups has 50 percent power.

However, given this depth of categorization of patients, it would be foolish to test the overall incidences of events, without taking patient categories into account. Medical knowledge would suggest that, at least for the placebo patients, increasing baseline severity should increase the probability of event and that smokers should have a higher probability of event. So any reasonable alternative hypothesis would have to include the possibility that the relative differences in probability of event between treatment and placebo would be affected by these two characteristics.

In designing a restricted significance test, the statistician would not know the exact probabilities of event (detailed earlier), but a restricted test can be constructed that is powerful against a general class of alternatives that would include this specific one. Thus, an appropriate restricted test will be one that takes the different severity classes and smoking status into account and is pointed at an alternative where the treatment might reduce the probability of event for the less severe classes and even reduce the relationship between baseline severity and probability of event.

On the other hand, the pharmacology of the agent being tested might suggest that the most dramatic differences will occur primarily in patients with the greatest untreated probabilities of event (the smokers and the most severe baselines). The point to be made is that any analysis of data like this should take into account the effects that seem reasonable from a prior knowledge of medicine and pharmacology.

How can this be done?

8.2. The Advantages of Blocking

When each patient's data are reduced to a Bernoulli variable (1 if event, 0 if no event), the potential statistical power to distinguish between treatment effects is reduced. We have to take advantage of the mathematical characteristics of the binomial distribution to restore some of that power by blocking the patients into relatively homogeneous groups. Once the patients are put into homogeneous blocks, the number of patients with events can be compared between treatments within each block. The occurrence of events are statistically independent from block to block, so the test statistics calculated within each block can be accumulated across blocks, and the accumulated test statistic has a known probability distribution, under the null hypothesis that the treatments have the same probabilities of event within block.

There are several ways in which these within-block test statistics can be accumulated across blocks. Suppose that

For each block, we compute a chi square test of the fit of the two frequencies to the null hypothesis that both treatments have the same probability of event.

Then, there are two methods of combining across blocks:

(1) Each of these chi squares has one degree of freedom. Since they are all independent, the sum of the chi squares is distributed as a chi square with degrees of freedom equal to the number of blocks.
(2) Tests across blocks can be calculated by separating the numerator and denominator of the individual chi squares, summing the signed square roots of the numerators and summing the denominators, and creating an overall chi square with one degree of freedom.

We can use either (1) or (2) for an overall significance test. Number (2) is the Mantel–Haenszel test (Mantel [1963]) and is most powerful against an alternative where the odds ratio of the two treatments is constant across blocks. Number (1) is most powerful where the major difference between treatments occurs in one or only a few of the blocks.

If the blocks have a natural order to them and if the difference between treatment is expected to be a monotone function of that order, test statistics such as the Armitage–Cochran test (Armitage[1955]) can be adapted to this problem. David [1947] found a test of the difference as a monotone function of order, which she called T. David's T is statistically independent of the chi square test (1), and she proposed combining these two tests to gain power against both types of alternatives.

To pick up the main theme of this book again, once the blocks have been established, a medically reasonable description of how the treatment effects might be expected to differ can be used to construct a class of alternative hypotheses. With such a class in hand, there are well-established statistical procedures that can be used to create significance tests that are powerful against those alternatives. But the starting point should be the medically reasonable description of what might be expected—not some arbitrarily chosen statistical procedure like Fisher's exact test.

8.3. Methods for Classifying Patients in Blocks

In general, there are three ways in which patients can be classified in blocks.

(1) Define the blocks in terms of baseline characteristics of the patients and define them in the protocol.

(2) Define the blocks in terms of baseline characteristics of the patients, but the blocks are defined after the study has been completed.
(3) Define the blocks in terms of events that occur during the course of the study (such as compliance).

From a purist point of view, method (1) leads to the fewest problems. The analyst cannot be accused of "data dredging" and finding a set of blocks that make the treatments appear different but that are a fortuitous combination of random noise. There is another advantage to defining the blocks in advance. It forces the study planners to think carefully about reasonable medical and pharmacological alternatives. In order for a blocking factor to be identified in advance, there has to be some reason to believe that patients with different characteristics (as defined by that factor) will respond differently to treatment.

Often, however, the large clinical study at hand is the first time data have been collected over a long enough period of time to determine that some baseline characteristics are important to the future course of the disease (and possibly to the way in which patients respond to active treatment). Under these circumstances, it is tempting to examine the outcome of the studies in order to find useful blocking factors. Factors found this way may appear to make sense in terms of the science. However, the analyst will be under a much greater obligation to show that they make sense than if the blocks had been defined in advance.

The reason for this general suspicion of blocks determined *ex post hoc* is that it is possible to find "blocks" that distort the true differences in treatment effect. This is especially true if the proportion of patients on a given treatment varies greatly from block to block. If the patients had been randomized to treatment, then severe imbalances are highly improbable. The justification of significance testing is that the observed treatment differences are highly improbable under the assumption of no treatment effect. However, the significance test only determines that a particular pattern of data or test statistic is improbable. If the test statistic is based on an improbable imbalance among treatments within block, a finding of "significance" may reflect that improbability rather than an improbability resulting from treatment effects.

However, "data dredging" is an honorable occupation. The statistical literature is filled with papers, in which the data at hand are used to define the mathematical model, which is then used to analyze the data. This is a method also widely used in science. It has disrepute only in the analysis of randomized controlled clinical trials. This is due primarily to the rigid approach to the design and analysis of RCTs that has become standard in the medical literature. There is nothing "evil" about using the data to define the model. The major problem is that we cannot be sure whether the model that has been found is "true" or is the result of one of Anscombe's Will o' the Wisps. For instance, the literature on discriminant analysis shows that discriminant functions do much better on the data set that was used to derive the parameters than on another data set generated out of the same distribution. But techniques have been developed that provide some protection against this type of error, and those who analyze clinical studies might consider them.

One simple technique is to separate the data into two sets at random. The first set is used to find useful baseline factors for blocking. The second set is used to test the hypothesis of no treatment differences, with the data blocked on the factors found in the first set. It has been my experience that it is useful to make the first set smaller than the second. Often, useful factors can be identified using only 10 percent of the data, so the second set (with 90 percent of the patients) retains adequate power to detect treatment differences.

Another method is known as cross-validation. In cross-validation, the data are broken into a large number of small equal-sized subsets (the subsets can be as small as a single patient.) The first subset is left out and the model is fit to the remaining patients. Then the fitted model is used to predict some aspect of the left-out subset and the deviation of what is observed in that subset from what was predicted is taken as a measure of how well the model fits. The sum of all the deviations, each one squared, is compared to the overall variance of the same measure across all patients. If the mean squared error (the average of the squared deviations) is considerably less than the variance (which is the mean squared error for a model that assumes all patients have the same mean), then the model is declared a good fit.

In the situation described in this chapter, each patient produces a (0, 1) variable of event/no event. Suppose we cross-validate using subsets of single patients. Then, with the ith patient left out, we divide the remaining patients into blocks and treatments (based on blocking factors identified after the study was complete) and assign the ith patient a probability of event, p_i, that occurs in the block and treatment to which that patient would have belonged. The discrepancy is, then,

$$(1 - p_i) \quad \text{if the event occurred in the } i\text{th patient}$$

$$(0 - p_i) \quad \text{if the event did not occur in the } i\text{th patient.}$$

The mean squared error is the average of these deviations squared. If the overall proportion of patients with event is $\mathbf{p}$, then the overall variance is

$$\mathbf{p}(1 - \mathbf{p})$$

and the mean squared error can be compared to this.

Finally, even if the blocks are identified after looking at the data, there is a way of determining the significance level that is unaffected by this sort of "data dredging." This is the permutation test. The use of permutation tests will be described in Chapter 9.

Up to this point, we have dealt with blocking factors defined by baseline characteristics of the patients. However, it is conceivable that events that occur after the study has begun will provide useful blocks of homogeneous patients. For instance, we usually collect compliance data (often in the form of returned pill counts). Compliance data is notoriously unreliable and often contains a great deal of missing data. And even if we knew exactly how many treatments the patient missed, it is still not clear how the analysis should be "adjusted" for that knowledge. However, it is possible to identify general classes of patients in terms of compliance. And those general classes can be used to block the analysis.

Compliance has been shown to be correlated with both placebo response and response to active medication (Hurwitz [1991]). This is probably because compliance does not necessarily affect response, but it is a surrogate for something that does affect response. A compliant patient will often be a patient who takes care of his or her health better than a noncompliant one. So compliance is a surrogate for attitude and action regarding ordinary preventive medicine. If we could identify patients by their neglect of general health, we might do better than with compliance. But we have compliance data and we do not have the other.

The statistical problem that arises if we block on events that occur after the study is underway is that the difference we find "significant" may be due to the treatment's affecting the blocking factor rather than due to the treatment's affecting the efficacy outcome. If the blocking factors are baseline measurements, then there is no way treatment could affect them, and a "significant" difference suggests treatment has an effect on outcome. But the use of post randomization blocking factors means that a "significant" difference between treatment groups may describe a difference in outcome, a difference in blocking factor, or a difference in both. However, a central theme of this book is that the initial overall significance test is a means of determining if there is enough information in the study to allow us to detect a difference between treatments. Once "significance" is found, the methods of estimation will be used to determine to what that significance is due. Because of this, it does not matter whether the "significant" effect is on the efficacy outcome, the blocking factor, or both. A finding of "significance" is adequate to start the examination of the data.

8.4. Trend Tests

If the blocks can be ordered and if we can expect a treatment effect to be related to that ordering, then the power of the significance test can be greatly improved by looking for a "trend." In general, let us indicate a sequence of blocks

$$B_1, B_2, B_3, \ldots, B_k$$

ordered so that the relative efficacy of the two treatments being tested increases with increasing block order.

Suppose that

X_{0i} = number of placebo patients in ith block who "respond,"

N_{0i} = total number of placebo patients in the ith block,

X_{1i} = number of treated patients in the ith block who "respond,"

N_{1i} = total number of treated patients in the ith block.

The angle transform can be used to convert these numbers into variables that are approximately normally distributed.

$$Y_{0i} = 2 \arcsin(\mathrm{sqrt}(X_{0i}/N_{0i})),$$

$$Y_{1i} = 2 \arcsin(\mathrm{sqrt}(X_{1i}/N_{1i})),$$

and then to the paired difference

$$Z_i = Y_{1i} - Y_{0i}, \quad \text{which has variance } (1/[N_{i1} - 3] + 1/[N_{0i} - 3]).$$

Under the null hypothesis of no treatment difference, all the Z_is have expectations of 0. A trend indicating alternative hypothesis would be

$$E(Z_i) = A + Bf(i), \quad \text{where } f(\ ) \text{ is some increasing function of } i.$$

The two parameters, A and B, can be estimated by least squares, and the log-likelihood ratio can be computed as

$$\sum_{i=1}^{k} \frac{Z_i^2 - (Z_i - [A + Bf(i)])^2}{\dfrac{1}{(N_{1i} - 3)} + \dfrac{1}{(N_{0i} - 3)}}.$$

This is also an example of Neyman's restricted chi square, and the test statistic is asymptotically distributed as a chi square with 2 degrees of freedom.

The preceding derivation leaves the function $f(\ )$ undefined. If the ordered blocks are based on some natural measurement of patient characteristics, such as the percent compliance, then $f(i)$ might be that measurement for the ith block. Data from previous studies might be used to model this function. However, the basic idea here is to increase the power of the significance test by taking advantage of an expected trend. So it is not necessary to model the trend function exactly. In fact, a simple use of the ordering indicator

$$f(i) = i$$

is often adequate to provide a powerful test.

Another use of ordering involves a modification of David's test (David [1947]). For each of the blocks, we can construct a chi squared test of the 2×2 table

X_{0i}	$N_{0i} - X_{0i}$
X_{1i}	$N_{1i} - X_{1i}$

David noted that the sum of these chi square tests will be powerful against an alternative hypothesis where one or more of the blocks has a large difference between treatments. To get at the subtle effects of ordering, David suggested an additional runs test based on the signs of the differences

$$X_{0i}/N_{0i} - X_{1i}/N_{1i}.$$

The runs test is statistically independent of the summed chi square test. so the two tests can be combined with a simple device. If

$$pc = \text{tail probability of the chi square test,}$$

$$pr = \text{tail probability of the runs test,}$$

then

$$-2\log_e(pc) - 2\log_e(pr)$$

is distributed as a chi square with four degrees of freedom, under the null hypothesis. David's test can be made even more powerful by doing the runs test on the signs of

$$U_i = (X_{0i}/N_{0i} - X_{1i}/N_{1i}) - (\textstyle\sum X_{0j}/\sum N_{0j} - \sum X_{1j}/\sum N_{1j}),$$

the deviations of the ith difference about the overall mean difference.

8.5. Weighted Categories

Once the patients have been divided into blocks of relatively homogeneous response patterns, then it becomes possible to address one difficult problem of interpretation that bedevils all controlled randomized trials. It is seldom mentioned in the discussion of such studies, but it has to be recognized that the patients who go into these studies are not "typical" of the patients who will benefit if the investigational treatment proves to be useful.

Epidemiologists have often confronted this problem. A sample of individuals may not resemble the appropriate population to which they will be compared. The epidemiologic solution is to create a set of weights

$$w_1, w_2, w_3, \ldots, w_k$$

that represent the relative strength each block has in the alternative (and more appropriate) population.

Similarly, in clinical studies we can construct values of w_i that give greater weight to blocks that occur more frequently in the overall patient population and less weight to blocks that occur less frequently. A properly weighted test statistic then is of the form

$$\textstyle\sum_i w_i T(X_{0i}, N_{0i}, X_{1i}, N_{1i}),$$

where $T(\ )$ is some test statistic (like the chi square) applied to the numbers of patients in each block. The theoretical distribution of this weighted test statistic can be determined since all its components are statistically independent.

This last description is less specific than the previous one, because it is not the intent of this book to lay out a sequence of recipes for analysis but to show how significance tests can be constructed, once careful thought has been given to what might be expected if there were treatment differences and to the circumstances toward which the study results will be extrapolated. Since the next step (after a finding of "significance") is to estimate the effects associated with treatment, it is worthwhile to consider weighted test statistics, which will provide such estimates directly.

CHAPTER 9

Permutation Tests and Resampling Techniques

9.1. Permutation Tests

Recall that in significance testing we observe data and propose as a null hypothesis a statistical model that could have generated such data, lacking a treatment effect. We then calculate the probability of the observed data. If that probability is very low, we conclude that the null hypothesis is inadequate to describe how the data were generated. To calculate the probability, we consider a set of possible observations:

The data we observed plus all possible patterns of data that would have been "more extreme" than these data.

The p-value we calculate is the probability (under the null hypothesis) of that entire set of possible observations.

We need to define what we mean by "more extreme," and the previous chapters were devoted to constructing alternative hypotheses that would define that concept. In general, we can think of that process as defining a test statistic, T, some number calculated out of the data from the different treatment groups, which is designed to increase in value as the data become more and more compatible with the alternative hypotheses. So, if we designate the value of the test statistic derived from the observed data by a lower case, t_o, and the possible random variable by the upper case T, then the p-value we calculate is simply

$$p = \text{Prob}\{T \geq t_o\}.$$

If we could enumerate all possible values of T, under the null hypothesis, and if each possible value was equally probable, then we could calculate the value of p by simply counting the number of possible values greater than or equal to t_o. This is the idea behind permutation tests.

For the study at hand, we randomly assigned patients to treatment. If the treatment did not have an effect, then the same probability distribution of the data would have occurred for any other random assignment of treatment. So, to run a permutation test, we calculate the value of the test statistic for the data, call it t_o. Then we reassign patients according to another randomization and calculate the test statistic, using the data observed from each patient but acting as if the patients had been assigned according to this other randomization. We do this for every possible randomization pattern. Since the randomizations were run independently of the treatment or the data, all possible randomization patterns were equally probable. So we need only count how many patterns lead to a value of the test statistic greater than or equal to t_o, the one generated by the original randomization.

Permutation tests were not really feasible before the advent of powerful and fast computers. Many theoretical papers appeared in the statistical literature during 1930 to 1960 showing how to approximate the permutation test p-value by the use of normal theory tests or nonparametric tests. By the 1990s, the computer allows us to count all permutations, and we can go directly to the exact calculation.

Computer programs that will perform permutation tests on widely used test statistics have been developed by Dallal [1988] and Mehta, Patel, and Sendchaudhur [1988a].

However, even with modern computers, a complete enumeration of all possible randomization patterns will take a long time. If there are 200 patients in the study, there are

$$2^{200} = 1.7 \times 10^{60}$$

possible patterns. It would take several days for a modern minicomputer to examine all of these.

There are two methods of coping with this problem. One is to generate several hundred thousand new randomization patterns at random and count those that have the test statistic sufficiently large. On the average, this procedure will produce the correct p-value with 95 percent confidence intervals that are less than ± 0.001 in width. Another method, described by Tukey [1989], views the initial randomization as consisting of two steps. In the first step, each clinic has a random sequence of symbols assigned, as

AABABBABBAABABAAB ....

In the second step, for each clinic, a random choice is made as to which treatment is assigned to which symbol. Then the number of randomization patterns that need to be enumerated can be restricted to those established by the second step. If there are 10 clinics, then there are

$$2^{10} = 1024$$

possible randomization patterns, a number small enough to be quickly enumerated on a computer but large enough to allow for significantly small p-values if there were true treatment differences. Other versions of permutation tests based on restricted randomization schemes can be found in Mehta, Patel, and Wei [1988b] and in Lachin [1988].

One important theoretical aspect of permutation tests is that the entire procedure is based on the possible reassignment of treatments and nothing else. *This means that the test statistic can be any combination of the data and that it need not be defined before examining the data.* The test statistic can be purely the result of "data dredging." When the p-value has to be calculated from a theoretical distribution of all possible experiments, then the test statistic has to be defined independently of the random fall of the data, since the random fall of the data is part of that theoretical distribution. However, any test statistic is independent of the enumeration of possible randomization patterns, so this problem no longer exists.

Thus, the use of permutation tests married to Neyman's concept of restricted tests produces a general procedure that is completely independent of the limitations of packaged computer programs and "standard" methods of statistical analysis:

(1) Describe, as completely as possible, the expected effects of treatment, using all the prior pharmacological and medical knowledge that went into the design of the study.
(2) Derive a test statistic that points at the expected effects. (If necessary, wait until the study is over to consider unexpected possible effects, in order to construct a test statistic that reflects both the prior knowledge and unexpected events that occurred during the trial.)
(3) Run a permutation test to determine the p-value associated with that test statistic's observed value or values more extreme.
(4) If the p-value is small, use the same test statistic to suggest confidence intervals on the effects of treatment.

The first three steps can be done within the framework of permutation tests. However, once we have a significant p-value, we have to assume that there is some effect due to treatment. In that case, the use of equally probable randomizations can provide us with no insight into the nature of that effect. Now, we need to model the probability distribution of the data, given that there is an effect.

9.2. Resampling

9.2.1. General Comments

To fix ideas, let us consider a study comparing a new antihypertensive drug to placebo. Significance testing has yielded evidence that the average drop in sitting diastolic blood pressure is greater for patients on the new drug than for patients on placebo. One of the medical questions to be answered now is one designed to be useful to the practicing physician:

If I prescribe this medication for a patient, how long should I wait before deciding that this particular patient is not going to respond to this drug?

One way to answer this question is to identify a subset of patients in the study who "respond." For each such patient, determine how long treatment had gone on before the patient's blood pressure dropped to the level defined as "response," then estimate an upper 90 percent tolerance bound on those times. In this way, we can answer the medical question with a statement of the form

90 *percent of all patients who respond will have responded by the end of* 4 *weeks, and* 50 *percent will have responded by the end of* 2 *weeks.*

But a direct naive estimate of this sort can be in error. Suppose we set "response" as a drop in diastolic blood pressure of 10 mm Hg or more, and suppose of the 60 patients randomized to treatment only 40 responded according to this definition. The 50th percentile is defined by 20 of these, and the 90th percentile is defined by the four patients who took the longest to "respond." Were we to run another study, it is quite likely that the 90th percentile would be a much different number. Ideally, we would like to treat a very large number of patients and estimate the 90th percentile of response time from all of them.

If the time to respond were normally distributed with a standard deviation of S, then we could use the average time to response and the standard deviation to compute upper 50 percent and 90 percent tolerance bounds. Or, if we knew the form of the probability distribution of time to response, we could use mathematical formulas derived from that distribution to calculate upper tolerance bounds. But we can never be sure of the "true" probability distribution of our estimators (especially in complicated situations involving conditioning variables, like this one).

The basic idea of resampling is that we use the observed data to generate an empirical probability distribution, which approximates the "true" but unknown one. We then use this empirical approximation to calculate confidence bounds or tolerance bounds.

9.2.2. The Jackknife

Suppose we are attempting to estimate the numerical answer to a specific medical or pharmacological question. For the moment, let us symbolize this unknown number as π. Suppose, also, that we can estimate the value of that number from the observed data as $\hat{\pi}$. (the symbol $\hat{}$ designates that the number has been estimated from the data). If X_i is the data from the ith patient, then we can think of a portion of the estimation due entirely to the randomness in X_i, symbolized as

$$Y_i = E(\hat{\pi} \mid X_i) = \text{expectation of } \hat{\pi}, \text{ given } X_i.$$

Since the only source of randomness in Y_i comes from X_i (all other contributions having been averaged out), the set of random variables

$$Y_1, Y_2, Y_3, \ldots, Y_n$$

is statistically independent, and we can calculate its average and standard deviation. If they are normally distributed, then we can even calculate confidence and tolerance bounds on π.

We can never really average out the contributions of all but the ith patient's data, but we can get a very close approximation to

$$E(\hat{\pi} \mid X_i).$$

Suppose $\hat{\pi}$ is the estimate using all n patients. Let us now leave out the ith patient and compute this estimate again, symbolized by

$$\hat{\pi}^i.$$

This is the estimate without the ith patient, so to a first-order approximation,

$$\hat{\pi}_i = n\hat{\pi} - (n - 1)\hat{\pi}^i$$

estimates the contribution of the ith patient to the original estimate. This estimated contribution, $\hat{\pi}_i$, is called the "pseudo-variate" estimate of π. Its expectation, conditional on X_i, is equal to

$$E(\hat{\pi} \mid X_i)$$

and the individual pseudovariates are asymptotically independent. As an added benefit, if $\hat{\pi}$ is biased, then the average of the pseudovariates is less biased. If

$$\tilde{\pi} = \sum \hat{\pi}_i/n,$$
$$S_j^2 = \sum (\hat{\pi}_i - \tilde{\pi})^2/(n - 1),$$

then $\tilde{\pi}$ and S_j can be treated as if they were the mean and sample standard deviation of a set of data, and t-tables can be used to compute confidence intervals on π.

The major problem with the jackknife (so-called because, like the boy's jackknife, it can be used as a general tool when nothing else is available) is that the true coverage of confidence intervals is not necessarily the nominal coverage. That is, if we compute a putative 95 percent confidence interval on π, the true probability of coverage may be more or less. If we view confidence bounds as a rough means of determining the difference between a 50:50 event and a nearly sure event, then the fact that nominal 95 percent coverage may mean only 80 percent coverage and that nominal 50 percent coverage may mean 60 percent coverage should not be too disturbing. However, there are examples where the nominal and true coverage differ by even more.

The problem with the jackknife's coverage seems due to the distribution of the pseudovariates, $\hat{\pi}_i$. If the pseudo-variates are symmetrically and smoothly distributed about their average, then the jackknifed confidence intervals tend to be close to correct in their coverage. But, if the pseudovariates are skewed in their distribution or tend to land on a small number of discrete values, then the true coverage may be considerably different from nominal.

One way to deal with this problem is to jackknife something slightly different from the direct answer to the original question. In general, if we wish to estimate some parameter, π, and there exists a monotone function $h(\ )$, such that we can also calculate

$$\beta = h(\pi),$$

then any probability statement about β can be converted into a probability statement about π since

$$\text{Prob}\{\beta \leq b\} = \text{Prob}\{\pi \leq h^{-1}(b)\}, \quad \text{where } h^{-1}(\ ) \text{ is the inverse of } h(\ ).$$

So, if we find a function $h(\ )$ that makes the pseudovariates more symmetric, we can be more sure of the coverage of the confidence interval. For instance, pseudovariates based directly on the Pearson product-moment correlation coefficient, r, tend to be skewed if the true correlation is not near 0.0, but the Fisher transformation

$$\beta = \text{arctanh}(r)/2$$

produces symmetrically distributed pseudovariates across all values of r.

Monte Carlo studies (Arvesen and Layard [1971], Arvesen and Salsburg [1973]) have shown that standard variance stabilizing transformations like

$\log_e$,
square root,
arcsin(sqrt),
arcsinh,
etc.

tend to produce more symmetric pseudovariates and more correct coverage for the confidence intervals that result.

If no symmetricising transformation seems available, there is a more general form of resampling.

9.2.3. The Bootstrap

Efron's bootstrap is a generalization of the jackknife (Efron [1982, 1987] and Efron and Tibshirani [1986]). DiCiccio and Romano [1985] have observed that there appear to be four reasons why the bootstrap has caught on in the statistical community:

(1) Elegance: like many of the best ideas in mathematics, the principle behind the bootstrap ... is simple and elegant, yet very powerful.

(2) Packaging: the catchy name "bootstrap" makes it easy for people to focus on the field ....
(3) Mathematical subtlety: There is sufficient complexity behind the bootstrap to lure the mathematical intellectuals on to the scene ....
(4) Ease of use: In contrast, for the practitioner, there is the hope of a fairly automatic and straightforward methodology that can be used without the need for any thought.

The jackknife allows us to use the variability seen in the data to estimate the underlying probability distribution that the random nature of the data induces on the parameter being estimated. It does so up to the second moment of that distribution. The bootstrap goes further. In some sense, all we know about the random nature of the observed data is the random fall of the data themselves. In fact, the observed data can be used to produce an empirical probability function, which is simply described as

$$\begin{aligned} &\text{Prob}\{X \le t\} \\ &\quad = (\text{number of observed values} \le t)/(\text{total number of observations}). \end{aligned}$$

A basic theorem of mathematical statistics (the Glivenko–Cantelli lemna, Loeve [1968]) states that this contains all the information in the data and that this empirical probability distribution is asymptotically equivalent to the true probability distribution.

To form the bootstrap, Efron proposed that we treat the empirical distribution function as if it were the true probability distribution function of the data. Then we can sample from that distribution to produce another set of data. From this randomly chosen second set of data we can compute the estimator again. We sample still again and get still another estimated value of π, and again and again, etc. In this way, we can get several thousand estimates of π.

If the initial estimate from the observed data is $\hat{\pi}$, and if the estimate from the jth random resample is $\hat{\pi}_j$, then we can order the thousands of differences

$$\hat{\pi} - \hat{\pi}_j,$$

and pick off the 5th and 95th percentiles. These can be used to form 90 percent confidence bounds about the true value of π. The Glivenko–Cantelli lemma guarantees that the coverage will be asymptotically correct.

What makes the bootstrap so enticing to the mathematicians is that we can add additional information to the empirical distribution function. We can modify it so that it allows us to sample a continuum of values (not just the ones we observed in the original data), if we believe that the data were generated by a continuous probability distribution. We can fold the empirical distribution function at its median, if we believe that the data were generated by a symmetric distribution. Efron has shown that, if we know that the data were generated by a specific family of distributions (such as the normal) and we force that onto the form of the empirical distribution function, then the bootstrap is exactly equivalent to the "standard" methods of computing confidence intervals, based on the known family of distributions.

For small sample sizes ($n < 30$), the bootstrap will sometimes produce biased answers (as occurs in many other small-sample procedures). To avoid the more severe problems, a number of modifications have been proposed, such as the bias corrected bootstrap and the accelerated bias-corrected bootstrap. Also, as in the case of the jackknife, a symmetricising transformation can improve the behavior of the method for small- to moderate-sized samples. However, most RCTs involve hundreds of patients, and the small sample problems are unimportant.

9.3. Afterthoughts

This chapter has been about freedom, the freedom to allow the data to suggest methods of analysis, the freedom to compute confidence intervals using subsets of the patients, and the freedom to propose a medically meaningful question without worrying about how that question might be answered within the framework of a statistical method. This freedom has come about because of the great power and speed of the modern computer. As statistical methodology moves into the 21st century, these methods of permutation tests and resampling will become more and more important. All these methods are conceptually quite simple, and computer programs to implement them are fairly easy to construct. However, as of this writing, very few of them have been incorporated into "standard" software.

Because of this lack of easily available software, the analyst who examines the results of an RCT may be forced to work within the "standard" system. However, it pays to know that all this freedom is just around the corner.

CHAPTER 10

Neyman's Restricted Chi Square Tests

10.1. Introduction

Throughout Neyman's papers, the idea of restricting significance tests to a well-defined class of alternative hypotheses keeps recurring. However, in one section of his work, the concept is not only made very explicit, but a technique for constructing restricted tests is derived. The work on restricted chi square tests appears in several papers by Neyman but is best summed up in a paper by Fix, Hodge, and Lehmann [1959].

Essential to an understanding of restricted chi square tests is the concept of the dimension of a hypothesis. A hypothesis about the distribution of a random variable can be thought of as a description of the probability distribution function. For instance, a binomially distributed random variable X, has a CDF of the form

$$\sum_{i=0}^{x} \binom{n}{i} p^i (1-p)^{(n-i)},$$

where the parameter, $\mathbf{p}$, is the (usually unknown) probability of event. We might be able to model the problem so that the probability of event, $\mathbf{p}$, is, itself a function of other parameters. For instance, in logistic regression, we observe covariates (like the patient's age), which we call Z, and we write the relationship between $\mathbf{p}$ and Z as

$$\log_e\left(\frac{p}{1-p}\right) = \alpha + \beta Z,$$

where the symbols α and β are parameters that are unknown and must be estimated from the data. If we combine the two formulas, we end up with a complicated expression, but it is really a function of two classes of numbers:

(1) the observed data, and
(2) the unknown parameters.

Once the RCT is completed, the observed data are available to us, so the complicated formula becomes a function only of the unknown parameters. That function can be described geometrically as a "surface" over a space, whose dimension is the number of parameters. Thus, in the logistic regression case, the CDF of the observed values of X can be thought of as a surface over a plane defined by α and β, which changes as we pick different values of α and β. Any other function of this probability distribution, such as Fisher's likelihood function, or a least-squares criterion of fit, can also be thought of as a surface over the α–β plane.

So, in Neyman's restricted test approach, we construct a probabilistic function of the data, which is a mathematical formula that includes a set of unknown parameters designated by letters. The number of free parameters, that is, parameters that are not assumed to be known but have to be estimated from the data, defines the dimension of the problem. If, in the case of logistic regression we wish to test whether age is a factor, we wish to test the null hypothesis that the parameter β is equal to zero. For, if β is zero, then age has no effect on the value of $\mathbf{p}$. So the null hypothesis consists of a space with one dimension, defined by the free parameter α and the alternative hypothesis consists of a space of two dimensions, defined by the pair of free parameters α and β.

10.2. Constructing a Restricted Test

In Neyman's general development, we compute the values of the data that would have been expected by a given model and the "distance" from what we did observe to what would have been expected. The statistic that tests a null hypothesis is the difference

Test statistic = Distance from observed data to the null hypothesis expectation − Distance from the observed data to the alternative hypothesis expectation.

Since the alternative hypothesis has more free parameters, its expectation is always closer to the observed data, and the test statistic is always positive.

There are two problems in constructing test statistics. One is to find a reasonably powerful test statistic that can distinguish between the null and alternative hypotheses. The other is determining the probability distribution of that test statistic under the null hypothesis, so we can determine the p-value associated with the test statistic. Neyman solved both problems explicitly for the case of a multidimensional contingency table and called it the "restricted chi square test."

In the most general sense, a contingency table results from categorizing patients according to several different criteria. Each category is a "cell" of the table, and we start by counting the number of patients who fall into each cell. The way in which the contingency table is displayed (columns = dose and rows = category of response, for instance) is a function of how well we expect the criteria of categorization to predict patient responses. We might assemble the cells by age, sex, initial severity of illness, and outcome. Or we might assemble the cells by dose of drug, race, and concommitant disease. Initially, however, it pays to think of the table as a long string of cells. Every patient is assigned to one and only one cell. If there are 300 cells in all, then the cells can be described in terms of 300 probabilities of assignment. Since the 300 probabilities have to add to 1.0, there are 299 free parameters that can be estimated from the data.

Thus, the most general alternative hypothesis is that all 299 probabilities are mathematically independent, and the "model" can be respresented as a point in a 299-dimensional simplex. A simplex is a space where all the values have to add to 1.0 and all are zero or positive. The best-fitting model is one that estimates the probabilities as

$$\text{Prob(Category } i)$$
$$= (\text{number of patients in category } i)/(\text{Total number of patients}).$$

The "distance" from the observed data to that best fitting-point is zero, regardless of how we define distance.

Suppose we have a more restricted model of the probabilities of categories. Suppose, for instance, we require that the numbers of patients in categories defined by dose be linear in dose. A linear function is defined by two parameters that have to be estimated, the intercept and the slope. Suppose there are five doses. We can subdivide the contingency table and replace every common grouping that contains the five doses by a two-parameter (rather than a five-parameter) model. Suppose the table is subdivided by sex, baseline severity (in four categories), and dose. The most general hypothesis involves

$$2(\text{sex}) \times 5(\text{doses}) \times 4(\text{severity}) - 1 = 39$$

free parameters. The restricted model with a linear dose response for each of the 8 (sex) × (severity) columns has

$$2(\text{sex}) \times 2(\text{linear dose}) \times 4(\text{severity}) - 1 = 15$$

free parameters.

Suppose, now, that we have a null hypothesis that the dose has no effect on category. Then the contingency table reduces to one without dose and has dimension

$$2(\text{sex}) \times 4(\text{severity}) - 1 = 7.$$

We can now compute two "distances," the "distance" from the observed data to the best-fitting alternative hypothesis in a 15-dimensional space and the "distance" from the observed data to the best-fitting null hypothesis in a 7-dimensional space.

10.3. Restricted Chi Square Tests

The "distances" just referred to are computed as chi square tests in Neyman's restricted chi square test methodology. That is, for each of the cells of the large contingency table we have two numbers

(1) the observed number of patients in that cell $= O_i$, and
(2) the expected number of patients (under some model) $= E_i$.

The "distance" is the sum

$$\sum_i \frac{(O_i - E_i)^2}{E_i}.$$

For a restricted chi square test, we compute this sum for the null hypothesis, and call it

$$\chi^2_{(s)}, \quad \text{where } s = \text{dimension of the null hypothesis space.}$$

We then compute this sum for the alternative hypothesis and call it

$$\chi^2_{(t)}, \quad \text{where } t = \text{dimension of the alternative hypothesis space.}$$

Since the null hypothesis is always nested within the alternative hypothesis, the dimensions are such that

$$s < t$$

and

$$\chi^2_{(t)} < \chi^2_{(s)}.$$

The restricted chi square test statistic is the difference

$$\chi^2_R = \chi^2_{(s)} - \chi^2_{(t)}.$$

It has the same probability distribution as a chi square with $(t - s)$ degrees of freedom.

10.4. An Example

Table 10.1 displays a two-dimensional contingency table, comparing the numbers of patients whose response is defined on a seven-point scale versus dose of drug. Has there been an effect due to drug?

A simple-minded approach is to propose the null hypothesis that the rows and columns are independent. The alternative is that the individual cells have

Table 10.1. Categories of Response Versus Dose

	Condition worse			No	Condition better		
Dose (mg)	Severe	Moderate	Slight	change	Slight	Moderate	Excellent
0	8	4	6	20	9	7	0
10	2	9	3	23	4	5	4
20	1	4	4	14	10	9	6
50	4	6	4	15	7	11	3

their own probabilities. We can approach this as a restricted chi square test by noting that, under the alternative, the expected number is equal to the observed for all cells, and that there are

$$7 \times 4 - 1 = 27$$

dimensions. So for the alternative hypothesis, we have

$$\chi^2_{(27)} = 0.$$

Under the null hypothesis (independent rows and columns), there are four possible probabilities for the doses and seven for the categories. But the four dose probabilities must add up to 1.0 and the seven category probabilities must also add to 1.0. So there are

$$3 + 6 = 9$$

dimensions. Under row and column indpendence, the probability for the i,jth cell is

$$p_{ij} = p_i p_j,$$

where p_i and p_j stand for the row and column probabilities. So with these to predict the values, we can compute a chi square distance from the null hypothesis

$$\chi^2_{(9)} = 25.19.$$

The restricted chi square test is then

$$\chi^2_R = 25.19 - 0.0 = 25.19,$$

which is distributed as a chi square with $27 - 9 = 18$ degrees of freedom.

The knowledgable reader will see that this is nothing but the usual chi square test for independence of rows and columns and that the degrees of freedom could also have been calculated as

$$(4 - 1) \times (7 - 1) = 18$$

the usual way. However, I have gone through this construction to show how the "standard" test fits into the broader framework of a restricted chi square test.

Note that the value 25.19 does not reach formal statistical significance. But the alternative hypothesis for this test was the general one of all possible patterns of cell probabilities. As noted in this book, we can gain a great deal by restricting the class of alternatives. In what follows, I will do so.

If the drug were working, then we would expect to see a dose response pattern. So, it makes sense to restrict the class of alternatives to those involving monotone dose responses. However, to use Neyman's formulation, we need to find a well-defined class with a definite dimension to the parameter space. There are tests against general monotone dose responses (see Barlow, Bartholomew, Bremner, and Brunk [1972]), but they cannot be fit into the restricted chi square scheme since they introduce dimensions that are random variables. There are a number of ways to introduce dose response. What follows is just one.

As a simple approximation of the expected monotone dose response, let us set the alternative hypothesis that

$$\text{Expectation}\{\text{category } i \mid \text{Dose}\} = \alpha_i + \beta_i\,(\text{dose}).$$

If the drug is "working," then we would expect that the slopes of these lines will go from negative for the worsening categories to positive for the improving categories.

Neyman showed that the asymptotic distributions of the restricted chi square test hold whether the parameters are estimated by minimum chi square, by least squares, or by maximum likelihood. So, using the standard least squares algorithms, we can estimate the parameters of the linear dose responses as follows:

Category	α	β
Deterioration:		
Severe	4.607	−0.043
Moderate	5.607	0.007
Slight	4.679	−0.021
No change	20.571	−0.129
Improvement		
Slight	7.643	0.000
Moderate	6.000	0.100
Excellent	2.536	0.036

These estimates suggest a drug effect, since the slopes start negative and end positive as we go from category to category. The chi squared "distance" from the observed data to this hypothesis is

$$\chi^2_{(14)} = 21.699$$

The dimension is 14 since there are two parameters for each of seven categories.

The null hypothesis of no drug effect that can be nested within this alternative is one for which all the slopes are 0.0. We then estimate the probability of category as constant and end with a "distance" of

$$\chi^2_{(7)} = 96.304.$$

This yields a restricted test of

$$\chi^2_R = 96.304 - 21.699 = 74.605,$$

distributed as a chi square with $14 - 7 = 7$ degrees of freedom. This has a p-value less than 0.001.

CHAPTER 11
Miscellaneous Methods for Increasing Power

11.1. General Principles

In the last five chapters, I tried to organize the use of restricted tests into general categories. However, there are too many techniques for strengthening power by paying attention to the class of reasonable alternatives to allow for a neat method of classification that covers them all. So, in what follows, I describe a mixed bag of additional "tricks" that a good analyst should have available.

11.2. Normal Theory Tests

When we assemble large sets of observations, there are very few examples of real data that truly follow a normal or Gaussian distribution. However, many of the most widely used significance tests are based on the assumption that the data are normally distributed. These include the t-tests (one- and two-sample), analysis of variance, and most tests based on the residuals from least squares regression. These are used because of "folk theorems" (widely held conjectures) that the p-values calculated from these tests are correct, even when the underlying distributions are not Gaussian. In less precise wording, normal theory tests are believed to be "robust."

Mathematical analyses like those due to Sheffe [1959] and Efron [1969] and extensive Monte Carlo studies (see Posten [1578], for example) have shown that at least two normal theory tests are, indeed, robust. These are the one-sample t-test and the one-way analysis of variance (which includes the two-sample t-test). To understand what this means we have to consider the two conditions under which one-way analysis of variance is run:

the null hypothesis that all the groups being compared come from the same normal distribution, with the same mean and variance.

the alternative that at least one of the groups being compared comes from a different distribution.

The "size" of the test is the phrase used to describe the true p-value of the observed data under the null hypothesis. As long as the "size" of a test is less than the nominal alpha level used to reject the null hypothesis, the test is "robust" for testing the null hypothesis. Suppose the patients are categorized

$$\begin{aligned} -3 &= \text{severe deterioration,} \\ -2 &= \text{moderate deterioration,} \\ -1 &= \text{mild deterioration,} \\ 0 &= \text{no change,} \\ 1 &= \text{mild improvement,} \\ 2 &= \text{moderate improvement,} \\ 3 &= \text{cure.} \end{aligned}$$

And suppose we decide to treat these scores as measures of response and run a two-sample t-test comparing the mean scores between a group of treated patients and a group of controls. Suppose, further, that the two-sample t-test yields a value of

$$t_{(28)} = 2.061.$$

If we look this up in a table of t-statistics, we will find that the nominal p-value is less than 0.025. Theoretical work by Efron and Monte Carlo studies suggests that the true p-value is less than 0.025, because the data come from a discrete rather than a continuous distribution.

But the other condition that may hold is the alternative hypothesis. We are interested in gaining the greatest power we can from the test, in order to detect a difference in distributions. By accepting a test that is "robust" in the sense that the true null-hypothesis p-value is less than the nominal one, we are also decreasing the power. (This is what lies at the heart of the controversy over use of Fisher's exact test when comparing two percentages. Fisher's exact test always has a true p-value less than or equal to the nominal one, thereby automatically decreasing the chance of detecting an effect, if there is one.)

We must now take a leap of faith (another folk theorem). We can investigate how slight modifications of the assumptions behind these tests will affect the power when the slight modifications still require that some of the data be

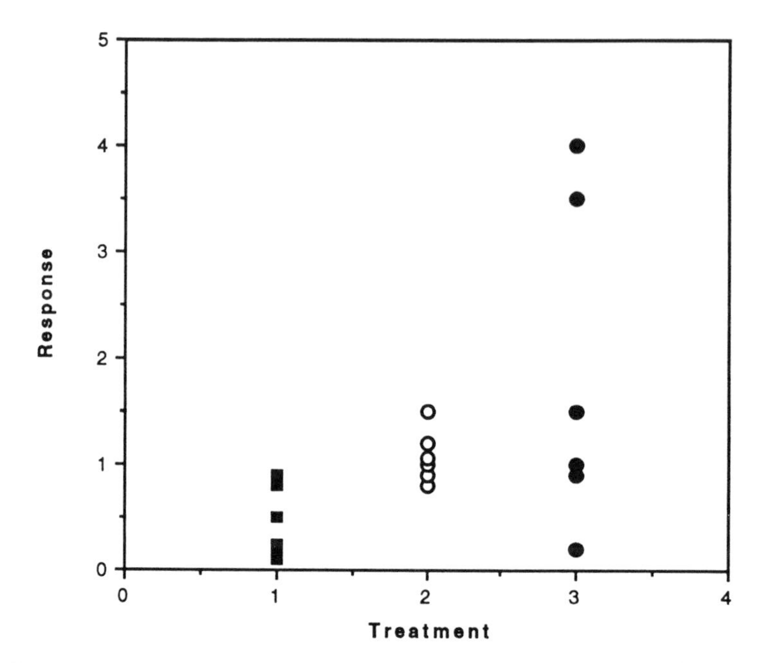

Figure 11.1. Responses to three treatments variance increasing with the mean.

normally distributed. The leap of faith is that these effects will also hold true when the data are not normally distributed.

11.2.1. Heterogeneity of Variance

One-way analysis of variance (and two-sample t-tests) are powerful against the alternative where each group is normally distributed with the same variance but where the means may differ. Suppose both the means and the variances differ. Under the null hypothesis, all groups come from the same distribution, so we can ignore the possible differences in variance, when it comes to constructing a valid test of the null. However, theoretical work by Sheffe has shown that if the variances differ, the test rapidly loses power. Intuitively, this is easy to see. Figure 11.1 displays the scatter of values for three treatments, where the variance increases with the mean. It can be seen that although the largest value in the third group is much greater than all the values in the first group, there are many values in the third group that fall within the range of the first group. If we assume that all groups have the same variance (remember, this is the null hypothesis, upon which the test statistic is based), the "best" estimate is the average of all the variances. So, the variance of the third group dominates, and the test statistic will tend to treat the difference among the means as well as within what would have been predicted by that variance.

There are two ways of modifying the test to take heterogeneity of variance into account. We can transform the data so that the variances are equal on the transformed scale. Or we can find an appropriate estimate of the variance (under the null hypothesis) that is not influenced by the heterogeneity.

11.2.2. Transformations of the Data

Suppose we measure some aspect of the patient's illness, like the time to walk 50 feet for a patient with osteoarthritis. Patients who have little disease will walk faster, and most of those with little disease will tend to walk at about the same rate. So, among patients who have improved, the walking time tends to have a small variance. However, patients whose hips or knees are giving them trouble will walk more slowly, and among these patients, there will be greater variability in the walking time. Thus, the measure will have a variance that increases with the mean.

There are many theoretical mathematical probability distributions, where the variance and the mean are related. If we knew the exact theoretical form of these measures, we could apply a formula from calculus that tells us exactly what transformation is needed to produce a measure on another scale, where the variance will be independent of the mean. It turns out that many of these variance-stabilizing transformations also tend to produce data that are closer to being normally distributed. Some examples are:

Distribution of X = measure	Transformation $Y = f(X)$
Binomial	$Y = \arcsin(\text{sqrt}(X))$
Poisson	$Y = \text{sqrt}(X)$
Sample correlation of 2 normals	$Y = \text{arctanh}(X)$

However, we seldom have the luxury of knowing the underlying distribution of our measure. So what is usually done is to collect groups of patients with similar values and plot the sample variance from each group against its average. The same formula from calculus lets us find the variance-stabilizing transformation if the relationship of variance to mean can be discerned from those plots.

If S^2 = sample variance and M = sample mean, then

$S^2 = g(M)$	$Y = f(X)$
$S^2 = M$	$Y = \text{sqrt}(X)$
$S^2 = M^2$	$Y = \log(X)$
$S^2 = M^4$	$Y = 1/X$.

One of these three transformations will often be adequate to stabilize the variance. Of course, if the original measurement is normally distributed, then the transformed value is not. However, the general null hypothesis robustness of the one-way ANOVA lets us treat the nominal p-values as appropriate. There are modifications to these transformations that attempt to adjust for situations that are not quite as straightforward. These can be found in papers by Freeman and Tukey [1950] and by Anscombe [1948].

Some practical problems of calculation and interpretation arise when using transformations. The problems of calculation occur when the original measurements have values that are undefined for the transformation. (There is no logarithm of zero or negative numbers, for instance.) Ad hoc procedures for handling these have been developed. When using the logarithm and there is a chance of getting a measurement of zero, the analyst will often add a small value to every measurement, so the transformation is

$$Y = \log(X + c), \quad \text{for some small number } c.$$

What value should be used for c? One choice is half the smallest nonzero value in the data set.

Since the square root will not take negative numbers, one procedure is to add a large value, C, to each measurement, large enough to be sure that no negative values remain.

Still another approach is to pick a transformation that behaves like the one we want when the data are in the defined range of the transformation we want, but that allows us to use data out of that defined range. A useful substitute for the logarithm is

$$Y = \text{arcsinh}(X) = \log(X + \text{sqrt}(X^2 + 1)).$$

If $X = 0$, then $Y = 0$. If X is negative, then Y is negative. If X is positive, then Y is positive.

The problems of interpretation are more difficult to overcome. Once the data have been transformed, the measurements of response are on a different scale. Sometimes it is relatively easy to interpret the new scale. For instance, if we use the log transform, then changes from baseline to final become equivalent to looking at the ratio of baseline to final, which can be easily converted to percent change. However, if we compare two treatment groups, using the log transform, then the comparison is not

$$(\text{percent change group I}) - (\text{Percent change group II})$$

but rather

$$\frac{(\text{Final value, Group I})/(\text{Baseline, Group I})}{(\text{Final value, Group II})/(\text{Baseline, Group II})}.$$

This ratio of ratios has no simple interpretation in terms of percent change from baseline. One method is to treat the significance test as an indicator that there is a difference between treatments and then use the intermediate data in the calculations to interpret that difference. If the log transformation has been used, one can construct confidence bounds on the percent change from baseline for each group, and these can be compared. Or, for any of these transformations, confidence intervals can be constructed on the mean of the transformed variable, Y, and those bounds converted back to the original scale.

For instance, if

$$Y_b \equiv \text{mean of sqrt(Baseline)},$$

$$Y_f = \text{mean of sqrt(Final)},$$

and if we use as measures of central tendency

$$X_b = Y_b^2,$$

$$X_f = Y_f^2,$$

then we can find $(X_f - X_b)$ an estimate of the change from final to baseline with the simple formula

$$(X_f - X_b) = (Y_f - Y_b)(Y_f + Y_b).$$

The same computation can be run if the symbols Y_f and Y_b stand for confidence bounds.

Similar reverse transformations can be found for other standard transformations.

11.2.3. Alternative Estimates of Variance

Under the null hypothesis, all the groups have the same variance. If the observed data indicate that the groups may have different variances, that, by itself, is an indication that the null hypothesis is not true. Thus, following the general principles laid down in Chapters 1 to 5, we could use a test for heterogeneity of variance and treat that as our one big significance test that tells us whether it is worth investigating the data further.

However, most of the available tests for heterogeneity of variance are not robust to the assumptions of normality. So a finding of "significance" may not necessarily tell us that the groups differ but rather that the data are not normally distributed. One test for differing variances that is not sensitive to assumptions of normality (since it makes no such assumptions) is the use of jackknifed pseudo-variates of the variance (Miller [1968]). Very little theoretical work has been done on the alternatives against which the jackknife is most powerful, so a failure to find significance using the jackknife may not be an appropriate signal that the data are not worth further investigation.

The fact that the null hypothesis assumes a constant variance (since it assumes that the treatment groups all have the same probability distribution) can help us here. The t-test for a two-sample problem and the F-test for a larger one-way ANOVA can be both thought of as a ratio

$$(\text{Scatter among means}) \div (\text{An estimate of the variance}).$$

The basic idea is that, if the null hypothesis is true, then the scatter among the means would be no greater than that predicted by the variance. The use of an F- or t-distribution results from recognizing that the denominator is an estimate of the true variance and thus is subject to random error. The larger the number of degrees of freedom associated with this estimate of the variance, the more precise is the denominator, and the calculations of p-values take this into account. However, the theory of these distributions does not dictate where the estimate of the variance has to come from. It is usually an estimate pooled from the several groups of the study under analysis. But it could have been taken from only one of the groups. Or it could be based entirely on data taken from a different study.

Thus, if there is reason to believe that the variances among the groups differ (due to changes in the means), then one can test the null hypothesis by using a valid, but small, estimate of the supposed constant variance. If the number of patients in the control group is 20 or more, we could simply use the sample variance from that group. Once we have 19 degrees of freedom (from $N = 20$), we gain little in the precision of the F- or t-test with the increases in degrees of freedom that might result from using the variance estimates of the other groups. On the other hand, if one or more of the treated groups has a high variance (due to an effect of treatment), including those estimates of variance in the denominator will most likely decrease the power. This whole question has been investigated in Brownie, Boos, and Hughes-Oliver [1990], where substantial increases in power are projected for this type of test under some circumstances.

11.3. Nonparametric Tests

11.3.1. General Principles

The general null hypothesis

H0: The probability distribution of data is independent of treatment

can be addressed by looking for a shift in the central tendency through use of the Wilcoxon rank sum test to compare two treatments or the Kruskal–Wallis ANOVA to compare three or more treatments. However, there are nonparametric tests that consider other aspects of the data.

If the distribution of the data is independent of treatment, then the random patterns of the data should not be affected by knowledge of the treatment assignments. The runs test (Fisz [1963]) orders all the data combined and counts the number of runs of consecutive values from the same treatment. If the random pattern is independent of treatment, then there should be a random pattern of run lengths and the distribution of the number of runs depends entirely on the number of patients in each treatment group. Other tests, like Tukey's quick test (Gans [1981]), examine the number of values from a given treatment that can be found among the extremes. Following the general principle of restricted tests, we should consider how the treatments might be expected to introduce patterns into the fall of the numbers and construct a nonparametric test that is sensitive to that type of pattern.

11.3.2. Testing For Heterogeneity of Variance

Differences in variance between two treatments can be addressed by procedures due to Ansari and Bradley, Moses, and Shorack (see Hollander and Wolfe [1973]). All of these make use of the fact that, if the treatments are all associated with the same variance, then the scatter away from the median should be the same. The Ansari-Bradley test, for instance, is a runs test applied to the absolute deviations from the overall median.

The fact that two treatments differ with respect to variance is hardly proof that one of the treatments has a "better" clinical effect than the other. However, as noted earlier, heterogeneity of variance is a warning that many standard tests will not be powerful, and a clear and obvious difference in variance should send the analyst to reexamining what might be expected clinically if the two treatments differed in effect.

11.3.3. Hajek Type Tests

When there is heterogeneity of variance, the situation cannot be "saved" by going to the standard nonparametric tests (Wilcoxon rank sum test for two samples or Kruskal–Wallis nonparametric one-way ANOVA). Noether [1967] has shown that these rank tests are very sensitive to heterogeneity of variance and rapidly lose power when this occurs. However, if the underlying cause of the heterogeneity can be identified, it might be possible to use a modified rank test of the class discussed by Hajek [1968]. An example can be found in Conover and Salsburg [1988].

The basic idea of the Hajek type test is that we model the alternative hypotheses in terms of a general probability transform. Suppose the measurement is one with a physiological bound beyond which it is not feasible to drive the patient. For instance, suppose we have an analog scale on which a patient indicates a degree of pain, the scale running from zero (no pain) to 50 (unbearable pain). It is clear that the maximum "improvement" possible on such a scale is 50. Without an effective treatment, we'd expect most patients to show an improvement, but the degree of improvement would tend to remain far from the upper bound of 50. So placebo-treated patients might have a symmetric distribution about some mean change (like 20). If the treatment is effective, then patients should tend to show a greater degree of improvement,

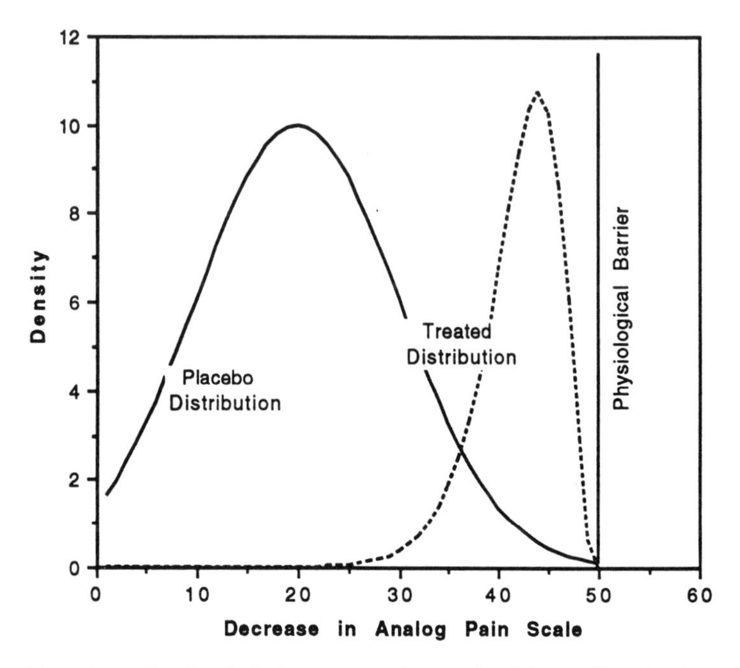

Figure 11.2. Example of a clinical measure where a physiological barrier bounds any possible improvement.

however, the maximum improvement of 50 creates a barrier against which the distribution of improvement scores will tend to pile up.

This sort of a situation is illustrated in Figure 11.2. The distribution for placebo is symmetric, but the distribution for the treated patients is skewed. In fact, if the mean difference tends to be small (due to a high placebo response), a statistical test of the mean differences will lack power, due to the skewness of the treated distribution.

We can conceive of the treated scores as representing the best of a set of placebo scores, so the piling up against the barrier is modeled:

H0: The distribution function for both placebo and treated is $F(t)$

H1: The distribution for placebo is $F(t)$, but for treated, it is $[F(t)]^k$ for some $k > 1$.

This is called a Lehmann alternative. We have introduced a parameter, k, which has a particular value ($k = 1$) under the null hypothesis, H0. However, the definition does not involve a specific mathematical model. The underlying distribution function, $F(t)$, is left undefined.

Hajek [1967] and Hajek and Sidak [1968] have a class of significance tests that cover such a situation. They are an extension of the more widely known nonparametric tests, such as the Wilcoxon and the normal scores test. With Hajek's method we can construct a test that is most powerful against the class of alternatives where k is close to 1.0. The idea is that if the test is most powerful where the effect is minimal, then it will tend to be powerful where the effect is even more.

In the case of a Lehmann alternative, the optimum test was developed earlier by I.R. Savage (see Hollander and Wolfe [1973]) and can be found in widely used software packages like SAS. However, Hajek's method of deriving locally most powerful tests can be applied to many other situations. Conover and Salsburg examined the case where the effect is a Lehmann alternative, but only a small percentage of the treated patients "respond." Johnson, Verrill, and Moore [1988] examined the case where the effect is a shift in the mean but only a small percentage of treated patients "respond." There is a simple mathematical method for deriving these tests, involving the first derivative of the density function. Once the alternative distribution can be modeled this way, a powerful nonparametric statistical test can be derived that is restricted to that class of alternatives. Use of this methodology awaits only the construction of medically meaningful classes of alternatives.

11.3.4. Generalized Thompson Tests

There is a generalized version of Hajek tests due to Thompson [1991]. To fix ideas, suppose we have observed T-4 cell counts on a group of ARCS patients (who have been randomized to four different regimens) at baseline, after 90 days, and after 180 days of treatment. Suppose, further, that these patients can be blocked at baseline by several different factors, such as T-4 cell count, use of AZT, and some measure of the opportunistic infections that have been seen in the past.

Thus, we have a very complicated design. Patients are divided in terms of

randomized treatment,
baseline T-4 level,
use of AZT, and
prior incidence of infection.

Within patient, there are three observations

0, 90, 180 days.

In Thompson's approach, we take all of the data and rank them, ignoring any of these subdivisions. We apply some Hajek-type transformation to the standardized ranks. And, finally, we locate a set of data that should have the same distribution under the null hypothesis of no treatment effect and that will have different distributions under the alternative. Coefficients are constructed that create linear combinations of the transformed ranks that are powerful against the expected alternatives. We can use one set of coefficients if there is a single well-defined alternative, or we can use more than one set if there are several possible alternatives.

Thompson derived the distribution of a test statistic based on these combinations of coefficients and Hajek transformation. The mathematics are easily computerized, and Thompson shows how to calculate the power of different sets of coefficients. Thus, Thompson tests provide a very flexible tool, which can start with a medical description of what is expected.

Using the example, suppose we expect that one of the treatments, if it works, will induce an increase in T-4 cell counts but that the increase will be greatest at 90 days and less so at 180 days. Suppose, further, that we would expect this to happen with greater probability in patients with the better prognosis, defined by the two baseline characteristics, and that the use of AZT may also have an effect. We can first choose a Hajek transformation that is most powerful against the type of statistical distribution we see in T-4 cell counts, increasing variance with decreasing value and a minimum value that some patients will achieve. Next we construct coefficients that allow for the change from 0 to 90 to be greater than the change from 90 to 180, that are adjusted for expected increases in effect depending upon blocks, and that sum to zero across treatments if there is no effect due to treatment.

I have been purposely vague about the exact Hajek transformation and the exact choice of coefficients. This is because I want to keep attention on the overall procedure and how it relates to medical expectations. However, a review of Thompson's work will show anyone with the mathematical knowledge to read it how these can be constructed.

CHAPTER 12
Bayesian Estimation

12.1. A Little Probability Theory

Suppose there are two events that can occur sometime in the future, which we will denote by the letters A and B. For instance, A might be the event that a patient will have his or her blood pressure lowered to "normal" by the treatment about to be given, and B is the event that the patient will remain free from stroke after five years of treatment. We can think of the events by themselves and talk about the probability of each, symbolized

$$\text{Prob}\{A\} \quad \text{and} \quad \text{Prob}\{B\},$$

or we can consider the probabilities associated with their relationship. Suppose we can lower the patient's blood pressure with treatment. Then we might expect that the probability of event B is different than if we had failed to lower the blood pressure. We might expect that the probability of event B, given that A has occurred, symbolized

$$\text{Prob}\{B \mid A\},$$

will be greater than unconditional $\text{Prob}\{B\}$.

But, once we have established a notation for conditional probability

$$\text{Prob}\{B \mid A\},$$

there is nothing to keep us from creating a symbol for the symmetric conditional probability of A, given B

$$\text{Prob}\{A \mid B\}$$

even though A occurs before B.

The Rev. Thomas Bayes appears to have been the first person to discover that there is a simple mathematical formula connecting these two symmetric symbols. But he refused to publish this result, since it clearly made no sense. If A occurs or does not occur before B can occur, how can one talk about the conditional probability of A, given B?

In spite of Bayes's misgivings, he prepared a monograph, and the monograph was published after his death. All his other works in theology and natural philosophy have become minor footnotes to history, unread and never thought of. But, this posthumous publication has made his fame (or notoriety). Furthermore, his name has been attached to a statistical heresy, because a portion of his formula is used to compute probability distributions about underlying parameters of other probability distributions.

The Bayesian heresy is simply stated:

Suppose that X is a random variable that can be observed.

Suppose, also, that the probabilities involved in values of X can be written in terms of a parameter π, so we have $\text{Prob}\{a < X \leq b \mid \pi\}$, *that is, the conditional probability that X will lie between a and b, given a fixed value of π. This conditional probability can be thought of as some function of π.*

Then,

we can propose that the parameter π is itself a random variable, and that it has a probability distribution, and that its probability distribution has parameters, $\beta 1$, $\beta 2$, ... βk, so that $\text{Prob}\{\pi \mid \beta 1, \beta 2, \ldots \beta k\}$ *is some function of the hyperparameters $\beta 1$, $\beta 2$, ... βk.*

Furthermore,

we can propose that each of the parameters of the probability distribution of π, the set of $\beta 1$, $\beta 2$, ..., βk, have probability distributions, with parameters.

And so on, infinitum.

The Bayesian heresy can be used with portions of Bayes's theorem to combine the observed data, X, with the prior distribution proposed for π to produce a posterior distribution of

$$\text{Prob}\{\pi \mid X\} = \text{probability associated with } \pi, \quad \text{given } X.$$

Thus, a Bayesian analysis of data consists of the sequence

$$\text{Prior on } \pi \rightarrow \text{Observed data} \rightarrow \text{Posterior on } \pi.$$

When the parameters of the prior distribution on π are themselves random variables with parameters, etc., the system is called a hierarchal Bayesian analysis.

Let us ignore, for the moment, where this prior distribution will come from or how to factor the hierarchal prior distribution into it. Instead, consider just the sequence from prior to data to posterior. Suppose that the prior distribution represents the scientist's strength of belief about the values of π.

For instance, suppose that we have a prior belief that reduction in blood pressure leads to a decrease in probability of stroke, and suppose we can quantify that belief so that the probability of being stroke-free after five years is a function of the blood pressure drop. In this model, π is the probability of being stroke-free. Its parameters are involved in the function of blood pressure that describes the probability of being stroke-free. To simplify matters, let us suppose that there are three types of patients

I. patients whose diastolic BPs drop to or below "normal,"
II. patients whose diastolic BPs do not drop to normal but do drop below 100 mm/Hg, and
III. patients whose diastolic BPs remain above 100 mm/Hg.

We can designate π_1 the probability of being stroke-free given event I, π_2 the probability of being stroke-free given event II, and π_3 the probability of being stroke-free given event III.

Suppose that the medical scientist approaches the results of a new study with some prior idea about the values of π_1, π_2, and π_3. He might be quite sure that

$$0.70 \leq \pi_1 \leq 0.99,$$
$$0.30 \leq \pi_2 \leq 0.75,$$
$$0 \leq \pi_3 \leq 0.25.$$

In the study at hand, suppose that we observe

$X_1 = 35$ out of the $N_1 = 50$ patients whose diastolic BPs are driven to "normal" who are stroke-free,

$X_2 = 10$ out of the $N_2 = 20$ patients with diastolic BPs above normal but less than 100 mm/Hg who are stroke-free,

$X_3 = 3$ out of the $N_3 = 3$ patients with diastolic BPs above 100 mm/Hg who are stroke-free.

Thus, 70 percent of the patients in group I remained stroke-free, very close to the lower limit expected, but well within what might be seen due to random noise if the true probability were higher. For patients in group II, the observed rate (50 percent) is in the range expected. For patients in group III, the observed rate (100 percent) is well above the range expected.

What can be done with such data?

The Bayesian analysis uses the observed data to modify the prior belief. For patients in group I, the stroke-free rate is at the lowest level expected, so the posterior distribution will force the scientist to reconsider and to produce a probability distribution that goes a little lower, in order to encompass this information. If the scientist has a very strong prior, then the occurrence of events that were not quite expected will not cause much of a shift. The most it will do is extend the range of probable values for π_1. That is, what was observed is a bit unexpected but not so surprising as to question the study, so henceforth the scientist must live with the possibility that keeping blood pressure at "normal" may not be as good at preventing stroke as previously believed.

What about group II? Here the results are just about where they were expected to be. So the data from the study strengthen the scientist's beliefs, and the posterior distribution should reflect this strengthening of belief.

Group III is a problem. The results (100 percent prevention) are beyond anything expected. The posterior distribution now becomes a compromise between the strength of belief described by the prior and the strength of the evidence. After all, 100 percent of the group III patients were stroke-free, but there were only three such patients. The posterior belief has to take into account the possibility that the stroke-free rate might be higher than thought before, but the bulk of the probability might still remain where it was because of the sparseness of the data.

This, then, is the Bayesian paradigm. We start with belief quantified as a probability distribution about some unobservable parameter (of the distribution of what we can observe). We observe, and then we modify our prior distribution based on what we observe. The statements that we make describe probabilities associated with the unobservable parameter. The probability distribution of the observed data plays only a passing role. We don't have to worry about problems of analyzing subsets of data or about keeping alpha-levels honest, or about the effects of sequential observations. All those problems go away. Furthermore we can now make statements like

I am 95 percent sure that the probability of being stroke-free after five years is greater than 50 percent.

or

There is a 50:50 *chance that the probability of being stroke-free after* 5 *years lies between* 80 *percent and* 95 *percent.*

The price of this freedom is the presentation of a prior. Is it a price you, the reader, are willing to pay?

12.2. The Arguments for Bayesian Analysis

The Bayesians point out that with a Bayesian analysis all mathematical tricks are "on the table." The observer can accept or reject the prior being presented. You can make your own prior. And others can examine the effects of modifying the prior on the final decisions. Bayesians claim that those who use frequentist calculations snatch criteria out of thin air. What does it mean, for instance, to talk about the tail probability of a distribution? The frequentists, they claim, will calculate a significance level by calculating the probability of what was observed plus anything more extreme. Why include in your calculations the probabilities of things that were not observed? the Bayesians ask.

If we consider how scientific decisions are made, the Bayesians point out, we can see that all scientists are acting as Bayesians. They approach each study with a prior mindset about what should be occurring. If what occurs is dramatically different from what they expect, they may reject the study, or they may slightly modify their prior mindset but not let the study results influence it very much, or they may redo the prior mindset completely. What they do depends upon the strength of prior belief and the strength of evidence in the study. How many times have randomized controlled clinical trials been described in published papers, where the authors go to great pains to dismiss some of the "findings" because they do not make "biological" or "medical" sense?

There is also a deep theoretical argument in favor of Bayesian analyses. This relates to the problem described in Chapter 3 of this book. If the patients who are recruited to a clinical trial are not representative of the patients to whom the results will be extrapolated, then it may turn out that statistical procedures that are optimum for any particular pattern of patient type will not be optimum if we wish to extrapolate the study results to another pattern of patient type. This problem is eliminated if the prior distribution includes probabilities about patterns of patient type. Under a Bayesian paradigm, there is an optimum procedure that holds for all possible patterns of patient type.

This ability of a Bayesian analysis to cut through a thicket of conflicting possibilities and produce a single optimum answer to any problem has made Bayesian analysis a widely used procedure in the theoretical statistical literature. No matter how complicated the problem, there is a Bayesian solution, so half or more of the articles appearing in journals like the *Annals of Statistics* make use of Bayesian calculations.

12.3. Neyman's Bayesian Derivation of Confidence Intervals

Jerzy Neyman could never be accused of the Bayesian heresy. He tried to force statistical practice into the theoretical structure of a frequentist interpretation of statistics. As indicated in Chapter 3, his attempt met with some serious inconsistencies, but it represents one of the most complete attempts to justify statistical practice within such an interpretation. However, he did take one excursion into Bayesian statistics. This was described in Chapter 4, but I review it here within the framework of a specific example.

We observe a random variable, X, which has a probability distribution based on a parameter, π. For any particular value of π, we can compute the central probability region on X

$$\text{Prob}\{a \leq X \leq b \mid \pi\} = 0.95,$$

where a and b are functions of π.

For instance, π might be the probability of being stroke-free after five years. If we watch 50 patients and $X =$ the number of patients who are stroke-free, then

$$\text{Prob}\{28 \leq X \leq 41 \mid \pi = 0.70\} = 0.95,$$

$$\text{Prob}\{31 \leq X \leq 44 \mid \pi = 0.75\} = 0.95,$$

$$\text{Prob}\{34 \leq X \leq 46 \mid \pi = 0.80\} = 0.95.$$

Suppose, he said, that Nature presents us with various possible values of π, depending upon the random events of the day. That is, there is no fixed and true value of π, but π itself is random with some probability distribution

$$\rho(\pi).$$

Let

$$T(\pi) = \text{Prob}\{a \leq X \leq b \mid \pi\}.$$

What is the average value of $T(\pi)$ as we allow π to range over its more or less probable values? If we rig things so that a and b are always chosen to make

$$T(\pi) = 0.95,$$

then, regardless of the distribution of π that nature throws at us, the average value has to be 0.95 (since it is always set equal to 0.95). This function $T(\pi)$ is Neyman's confidence interval. Thus, if we construct a confidence interval on π, Neyman said we will know that the average "coverage" of the interval will be 0.95.

In this derivation, Neyman did not attempt to convert the mathematical concept of average "coverage" to something with a real-life interpretation. So this derivation can be taken as an empty exercise in cute mathematics. On the other hand, if we can ascribe a real-life meaning to average "coverage," then this derivation allows us to compute confidence intervals based on subsets of patients, without worrying about the multiplicity problem. To see why this is, let the probability distribution of π be conditional upon the choice of subset of patient. The same proof goes through and the average "coverage" is as advertised.

All we need is a real-life interpretation of the average "coverage." One possible interpretation is one that falls within the Bayesian paradigm of

$$\text{prior} \rightarrow \text{observations} \rightarrow \text{posterior}.$$

The posterior provides a 95 percent region of belief about the parameter, after the data have been observed, sometimes called a credibility region. If we begin with a specific prior distribution, we can compute the 95 percent credibility region. But, according to Neyman's proof, we can consider another region. This is a region of values for π that will average 95 percent probability, regardless of what prior distribution has been chosen. Neyman's proof stops just short of computing the posterior distribution and considers ranges of probable observations in terms of the prior. If the parameter being estimated is a measure of central tendency, like the mean or the median, then the 95 percent credibility region comes very close to the 95 percent confidence interval. With a little careful mathematics, we can always reformulate the problem at hand so that we have a probability distribution, for which the parameter being estimated is the central tendency. Thus, if we do not want to invest in a specific prior, we can use Neyman's confidence intervals as reasonably good approximations of the Bayesian posterior credibility regions.

Another justification for using confidence intervals as approximations of Bayesian posterior credibility regions is what Savage [1961] called the likelihood principle. When computing the posterior distribution with a large amount of data, it turns out that the central region of the posterior distribution is not much affected by the prior. Instead, the central region of the posterior resembles the likelihood function of the data. So credibility regions that do not go too far into the extremes can be approximated by confidence intervals based on the likelihood function. Most of the standard test statistics used to compute confidence intervals are monotone functions of the likelihood, which means that Savage's likelihood principle allows us to use these confidence intervals. How wide can we make the confidence region before we get into the tails of the posterior and have to take the prior into account? That depends, of course, on the shape of the likelihood and the amount of data. But with the sample sizes we use in RCTs, we can be probably go as high as 95 percent.

Thus, the Bayesian paradigm, along with the likelihood principle and Neyman's first proof, allows us to do something that the frequentists view with horror and that is violently denounced in most standard statistics textbooks. We can, in fact, take 50 percent and 95 percent confidence intervals and make statements like

I am 50 *percent sure that the true value of the parameter lies within this range.*

There is a 95 *percent probability that the parameter lies between....*

12.4. What Can Be Calculated and What Cannot?

Bayesian analysis has no place for significance tests as such. There is no direct link between the tail probability of a significance test and anything that can be calculated under the Bayesian paradigm. However, as noted earlier, Bayesian analysis allows the scientist to make the type of statement that the naive user of significance tests and confidence intervals is often tempted to make, statements like

The probability that the null hypothesis is true is less than 0.05.
The probability that the alternative is more true than the null is 0.95.
The odds in favor of the alternative are 20:80.

Suppose we have a parameter π. The null hypothesis is a statement about the parameter π.

$$\text{H0: } a \leq \pi \leq b$$

And the alternative is also a statement about the parameter π.

$$\text{H1: } b < c \leq \pi$$

For instance, suppose π is the probability of being stroke-free at five years. The null hypothesis might be that π is less than 0.50

$$\text{H0: } 0 \leq \pi \leq 0.50.$$

While the alternative might be that π is greater than 0.75,

$$\text{H1: } 0.50 < 0.75 \leq \pi \leq 1.00.$$

We can now make a Bayesian statement about the relative probability of H0 or H1.

However, trying to force a Bayesian analysis into the straitjacket of hypothesis testing is a rather foolish tour-de-force. The important aspect of Bayesian analysis is that it provides an entirely different view of the methods of statistical analysis. This is the ability to make a probability statement about a region of interest for a given parameter. Thus, the best use of Bayesian analysis in a clinical study would be to provide an alternative to the computation of confidence interval—an alternative whose real-life interpretation is straightforward.

There are two mathematically simple versions of Bayesian analyses that are easy to use and that take advantage of the concept of a conjugate prior.

12.4.1. The Mean of a Normal Distribution

Let X be a normally distributed random variable with

$$\text{mean} = m,$$

$$\text{variance} = S^2.$$

Suppose that the mean, m, has a prior normal distribution with its

$$\text{mean} = \mu,$$

$$\text{variance} = \tau^2.$$

Then the posterior distribution on m is also normal, with

$$\text{mean} = (\tau^2 X + S^2\mu)/(S^2 + \tau^2),$$
$$\text{variance} = (S^2\tau^2)/(S^2 + \tau^2).$$

[One practical problem with this formulation is that we do not know the true value of the variance of X, but we can estimate it from the data. When we estimate it from the data, there are slight modifications that have to be made to these formulas (see Morris [1983]). However, for clinical studies with 30 or more patients, these modifications have little effect on the final calculations, so they can be ignored.]

Suppose, as an example, we have a study comparing two antihypertensive agents and X is the average difference in drop in diastolic BP. Then S^2 can be calculated from the standard error of the mean difference. Where can we get μ and τ^2 from? These are easily computed by asking the scientist to give a range of values she is "sure" the true mean will fall between. This range of values can be taken as the 95 percent probability region of the prior. Their midpoint is the value of μ, and one-fourth their difference is an estimate of τ.

12.4.2. The Probability of a Binomial Distribution

If p is the probability of a binomial distribution and we observe X out of n patients who "respond," then there is a conjugate prior Bayesian formula. The conjugate prior requires that p has a beta distribution. The beta distribution has two parameters, α and β, but we can think of these parameters as having the following relationship

$\alpha/(\alpha + \beta)$ is the best prior estimate of the mean value of p,

$(\alpha + \beta)$ represents how sure the analyst is of that value of p.

The sureness of that choice of p can be thought of in terms of a hypothetical trial that might have taken place prior to this one. The value of $(\alpha + \beta)$ is equivalent to the sample size of that trial. Thus, the analyst might state that he estimates that the mean is 0.75 and that he is as sure of this as if he had observed 100 patients and found 75 of them "responding."

On another level, the parameters α and β of the prior can be elicited by asking the analyst to supply a mean value for p and a 95 percent range. The values of α and β can be computed from tables of the incomplete beta function.

Suppose, now, that we observe X out of n "responders." The posterior distribution on p is also a beta with parameters

$$\alpha' = \alpha + X,$$
$$\beta' = \beta + n - X.$$

Posterior probability regions can be computed from the incomplete beta function. A simple approximation is the following from Abramowitz and Stegun [1964].

Let

$$q = (\alpha + \beta - 1)(1 - x)(3 - x) - (1 - x)(\beta - 1),$$
$$v = 2\beta,$$

then if P has a beta distribution with parameters α and β,

$$\text{Prob}\{P \leq x\} = \text{Prob}\{Z \leq q\},$$

where

Z has a chi square distribution with v degrees of freedom.

12.5. Empirical Bayes Procedures

One modification of the Bayesian paradigm due to Robbins [1964] takes the position that we have a series of experiments and that the underlying parameter, π, is different for each experiment. The results of the series of experiments can then be used to construct a "prior" distribution on the parameter. This "prior" distribution is, in fact, a potentially observable random event, so the likelihood function can be modified to include the distribution of π and the hyperparameters of that distribution can be estimated by maximum likelihood.

In Robbins' original formulation of empirical Bayes, he used clever mathematical manipulations to find estimators of the underlying parameters of the Bayesian prior that could be calculated from the data directly. Morris [1983] expanded Robbins' specific examples into a more general framework, where the parameter π and the parameters of its distribution are all part of the formula. Copas [1972], taking a different tack, developed general methods for estimating the underlying mean and variance of the parameter π. Using Morris' formulation, we get estimators of the underlying parameters and fit them into the parametric model. Using Copas' formulation, we act as if the parameter π is normally distributed and compute its distribution from the mean and variance. What should be clear from this paragraph is that the concept of empirical Bayes is not well-defined and that there are several methods of analysis that can be called "empirical Bayes."

If the design of the current trial is sufficiently complex (with different identifiable subsets of patients). then we do not even need a sequence of prior trials, but we can estimate the hyperparameters directly from the data of the current trial. A classic example of this is described in Hui and Berger [1983], where a large group of women of varying ages were followed for periods of 3 to 10 years with annual measurements made of bone mass. The rate of change was taken as the parameter of interest. It was assumed, in turn, that this parameter was normally distributed but linearly related to age. And the hyperparameters of that linear relationship were estimated from the combined prior/current data likelihood function.

12.6. The Role of Bayesian Methods in Clinical Research

This heading has been the topic of books (see O'Hagan [1988] and Savage [1954] for examples), and there are persuasive arguments that can be made for throwing out the entire paraphernalia of significance tests and frequentist interpretations and resting all analyses on the Bayesian paradigm. An excellent discussion of the Bayesian view toward clinical studies can be found in Breslow [1990]. In this book, I have taken an intermediate position. I recognize that the frequentist interpretation and the Neyman–Pearson formulation of hypothesis testing are philosophically untenable. But I also recognize the need for a clear "objective" means of determining the difference between events that are medically meaningful and those that are the results of mere random noise. So I have taken the position that the first step in the analysis of a clinical study is a single overall significance test to determine if the study provides evidence of a "signal" in the midst of the noise.

However, once the overall significance test has shown that there is a detectable signal, then Bayesian procedures may prove very useful in determining the nature of that signal. As I have shown earlier, I think that the next step is the construction of interval estimates of answers to highly specific medical questions. These estimates should fulfill the following minimum requirements:

(1) Their width should increase with increasing uncertainty, whether that uncertainty is due to the small number of patients involved or to a wide range of results for those patients.
(2) The estimates should enable us to distinguish between ranges of answers that are "quite sure," those that are "50:50," and those that are "in between."

The machinery of Neyman confidence intervals provides us with interval estimates that meet both of these requirements. But so do the tools of Bayesian analysis. The two methods of calculation will seldom produce exactly the same numerical answers, but as shown earlier in the discussion of the likelihood principle, they should produce answers that are similar.

CHAPTER 13
An Example of the Type of Analysis Suggested in This Book

13.1. The Study

In this chapter I describe a statistical analysis of a single study that uses the principles and some of the techniques described in earlier chapters. The study is a two-center study comparing patients with clinical depression between two treatments:

Treatment A = a dibenzoxepin derivative,

Treatment B = a combination of amitriptyline and a phenothiazine.

Patients were screened to meet entrance criteria, randomized to treatment, and treated for eight weeks as outpatients, with clinic visits at

Baseline (just before randomization),
Week 2 of treatment,
Week 4 of treatment,
Week 6 of treatment, and
Week 8 of treatment.

At each of these clinic visits, the patients were evaluated using the Hamilton Depression Scale. The Hamilton Depression Scale consists of 17 items, rated with values 1 to 4, with 1 the least severe and 4 the most severe. Each item describes highly specific symptoms or behavior patterns. The rater is asked to concentrate on a given item, ignoring any interrelationship with other symptoms, and to grade that item in isolation. The clinical meaning of each graded value is described in great detail to standardize the use of the instrument across raters.

The vector of 17 item-scores has been factor-analyzed using different patient populations, and four factors have emerged that are stable across patient

Table 13.1. Hamilton Depression Scale Factors

Number	Factor name	Most heavily weighted items
I	Anxiety/somatization	Anxiety, psychic
		Anxiety, somatic
		G-I somatic symptoms
		General somatic symptoms
		Hypochondriasis
		Lack of insight
II	Cognitive disturbance	Feelings of guilt
		Suicide
		Agitation
		Depersonalization and derealization
III	Retardation	Depressed mood
		Work and activities
		Retardation
		Genital symptoms
IV	Sleep disturbance	Insomnia, early
		Insomnia, middle
		Insomnia, late

type, rater, sex, and nationality. Each factor is a weighted sum of the 17 items. The mathematical theories behind factor analysis show that the individual factors are uncorrelated with each other. That is, the fact that a patient has a particular value on factor 1, for instance, provides no additional information for predicting that patient's value on factor 2, or factor 3, or factor 4. This independence of the factors will play an important role in the analysis of the data. The factors are described in Table 13.1. The data to be analyzed in this chapter consist of the four factor values at each visit for each patient.

There are some added complications to the data. Although the protocol called for patients to be treated for eight weeks, 21 of the 65 patients in the study (32.3 percent) dropped out before the end. Most of these patients were dropped by the investigators because of a lack of efficacy. One patient failed to return after the baseline visit and could not be located.

Table 13.2 displays the raw data for this analysis, the values of the four factors at each visit for each patient. There were two centers. Each center used a separate randomization list. The numbers of patients enrolled were as follows:

	Treatment	
Center	A	B
20	16	13
4	18	15

Table 13.2. Hamilton Depression Scale Factor Scores

				HAMD factors			
Center	Patient	Treatment	Week	1	2	3	4
20	1	B	1	11.628	7.516	3.663	2.344
			2	6.591	5.217	3.906	1.346
			3	6.014	7.906	3.208	1.691
			4	6.014	7.906	3.208	1.691
			5	6.014	7.906	3.208	1.691
20	2	B	1	11.059	7.651	4.812	2.114
			2	11.491	7.976	4.847	2.506
			3	12.089	7.004	3.994	2.792
			4	14.762	7.458	5.472	2.968
20	3	B	1	11.439	8.216	5.075	2.304
			2	13.229	6.921	5.014	3.294
			3	8.407	7.864	3.372	2.670
			4	9.110	8.510	3.807	2.456
			5	9.110	8.510	3.807	2.456
20	4	B	1	11.422	6.455	4.012	2.896
			2	12.148	6.573	4.256	2.380
			3	9.937	7.028	2.959	3.047
			4	11.070	6.158	4.109	2.932
			5	11.021	6.825	3.374	1.632
20	5	B	1	9.676	7.518	2.529	2.098
20	6	B	1	11.442	6.426	5.110	3.865
			2	8.614	5.855	3.520	2.652
			3	8.017	5.087	3.068	2.454
			4	5.544	7.114	3.625	1.486
			5	5.544	7.114	3.625	1.486
20	7	B	1	11.743	7.082	4.360	3.110
			2	11.087	7.656	3.941	2.953
20	8	B	1	12.275	7.078	3.687	2.291
			2	14.165	6.839	4.825	2.356
20	9	B	1	12.770	7.068	4.176	2.572
			2	9.193	6.924	2.625	1.868
			3	10.968	7.965	4.441	2.662
20	10	B	1	10.683	6.454	3.678	1.972
			2	4.549	0.995	0.370	0.397
			3	4.549	0.995	0.370	0.397
			4	4.549	0.995	0.370	0.397
			5	4.549	0.995	0.370	0.397
20	11	B	1	11.330	7.807	3.451	2.620
			2	12.888	8.417	4.484	2.403

Table 13.2 (cont.)

Center	Patient	Treatment	Week	HAMD factors 1	2	3	4
			3	12.812	7.990	4.563	2.698
			4	8.560	5.963	3.711	2.258
			5	8.560	5.963	3.711	2.258
20	12	A	1	13.740	6.609	3.469	2.634
			2	10.932	7.514	3.850	2.343
			3	10.317	6.872	3.690	2.621
			4	7.755	5.693	2.186	2.823
			5	7.664	4.648	2.854	2.646
20	13	A	1	12.378	6.971	3.700	2.718
			2	11.975	7.221	4.180	3.139
			3	11.032	7.037	5.221	3.552
20	14	B	1	13.052	7.172	4.430	2.463
			2	12.130	7.246	3.526	2.330
			3	9.952	5.602	3.316	1.764
			4	10.237	5.874	3.980	2.053
			5	12.855	7.017	4.372	2.723
20	15	A	1	11.575	7.783	4.977	3.199
20	16	A	1	11.871	5.784	5.892	2.208
			2	10.811	7.598	4.324	2.806
			3	11.391	6.950	3.190	2.361
			4	11.626	6.621	3.892	2.108
			5	6.561	5.265	3.225	1.538
20	17	A	1	12.057	8.468	4.998	2.208
			2	9.723	7.452	4.317	3.101
			3	8.509	7.004	3.682	2.149
			4	5.941	6.965	3.022	1.729
20	18	A	1	11.999	9.346	4.282	2.417
			2	10.710	7.685	3.959	2.963
			3	8.121	6.556	3.874	2.089
			4	6.377	5.900	4.144	0.955
20	19	A	1	11.845	7.576	4.358	2.466
			2	11.321	7.068	3.832	1.823
			3	12.218	7.250	3.801	2.394
			4	7.587	6.902	1.851	2.744
20	20	B	1	10.836	7.260	4.206	2.680
			2	11.794	3.331	2.609	2.648
			3	8.542	7.776	3.278	2.377
			4	8.832	8.192	4.630	2.615
20	21	A	1	12.123	7.566	5.544	2.705

Table 13.2 (cont.)

Center	Patient	Treatment	Week	HAMD factors 1	2	3	4
20	22	A	1	12.767	7.714	4.394	2.104
			2	11.950	7.412	4.187	2.524
			3	9.088	7.403	3.192	2.522
			4	11.140	4.816	4.260	2.202
20	23	A	1	12.359	7.537	4.221	2.771
			2	12.540	7.171	4.734	2.517
			3	12.105	5.395	2.700	3.058
			4	11.077	7.346	4.011	2.304
			5	9.169	6.514	2.647	2.324
20	24	A	1	10.775	7.147	3.733	2.487
			2	11.866	6.953	3.653	2.044
			3	9.844	7.592	2.926	1.909
			4	9.901	7.420	2.812	1.806
			5	9.901	7.420	2.812	1.806
20	25	A	1	11.511	8.189	4.680	2.679
			2	11.511	8.189	4.680	2.679
			3	11.806	6.971	3.211	2.455
			4	12.642	8.087	4.439	3.471
			5	10.051	8.057	2.913	2.298
20	26	A	1	13.351	7.985	5.384	2.882
			2	12.346	7.189	4.564	2.937
			3	9.826	8.703	3.209	1.940
			4	9.826	8.703	3.209	1.940
			5	8.192	6.740	2.739	2.697
20	27	A	1	10.458	7.653	3.453	2.118
			2	11.828	7.683	4.960	3.048
20	28	A	1	10.129	7.898	3.806	2.308
			2	7.608	6.933	3.723	3.127
			3	7.341	5.856	4.068	2.078
			4	8.121	6.501	3.987	2.229
			5	6.763	5.482	3.167	3.356
20	29	A	1	10.650	6.840	4.245	2.353
			2	10.458	7.653	3.453	2.118
			3	12.096	6.643	4.363	3.556
			4	8.383	6.104	2.827	1.836
			5	8.383	6.104	2.827	1.836
4	30	A	1	14.940	9.554	6.303	2.403
			2	9.647	5.525	2.381	0.891
			3	8.840	4.802	2.748	0.483
			4	5.972	4.743	2.002	0.385
			5	13.740	6.555	4.001	2.273

Table 13.2 (cont.)

Center	Patient	Treatment	Week	HAMD factors 1	2	3	4
4	101	A	1	10.544	9.830	5.002	2.370
			2	9.238	5.897	3.630	1.700
			3	7.195	4.490	1.192	1.092
			4	5.209	4.080	0.935	1.563
			5	6.389	4.990	2.152	1.934
4	102	A	1	12.511	8.729	6.364	3.886
			2	10.720	7.067	4.023	2.153
			3	6.455	4.237	2.326	1.584
			4	5.827	4.712	5.589	2.288
			5	10.790	6.648	3.885	2.934
4	103	A	1	12.944	8.298	3.944	1.535
			2	5.097	4.314	2.345	2.256
			3	5.803	5.192	2.773	1.872
4	104	A	1	8.027	6.891	1.890	1.671
			2	6.471	7.983	4.048	1.246
			3	6.628	8.350	4.165	1.102
			4	9.474	8.567	3.053	1.319
			5	9.847	8.241	2.496	1.247
4	105	A	1	9.732	10.291	3.976	1.892
			2	9.732	10.291	3.976	1.892
4	106	A	1	9.264	6.686	4.707	2.657
			2	9.264	6.686	4.707	2.657
			3	5.959	5.451	3.040	2.380
			4	5.344	4.809	2.880	2.658
			5	9.264	6.686	4.707	2.657
4	107	A	1	13.198	10.331	3.782	2.373
			2	10.564	9.400	3.436	2.727
			3	8.460	6.463	2.432	2.322
			4	5.670	4.544	1.724	0.568
			5	5.212	4.269	1.681	0.702
4	108	A	1	12.311	8.874	2.663	2.666
			2	12.311	8.874	2.663	2.666
			3	12.311	8.874	2.663	2.666
4	109	A	1	14.913	9.139	3.809	1.981
			2	10.059	8.157	2.883	1.947
			3	6.315	4.847	2.495	0.925
4	9	B	1	12.805	6.753	4.792	1.750
			2	10.672	5.877	3.971	1.279
			3	8.855	4.870	3.266	0.631
			4	15.855	7.859	4.093	3.005

Table 13.2 (cont.)

				HAMD factors			
Center	Patient	Treatment	Week	1	2	3	4
4	10	B	1	11.471	9.870	4.956	2.140
			2	10.035	7.931	5.653	2.045
			3	11.071	10.821	4.141	3.605
4	110	A	1	13.206	9.233	5.822	2.152
			2	7.362	5.580	3.066	2.633
			3	5.627	4.355	1.905	2.040
			4	5.315	5.010	2.538	1.169
			5	6.806	4.682	2.982	1.182
4	111	A	1	14.950	8.202	3.851	2.609
			2	10.333	6.657	2.906	1.922
			3	7.242	4.669	2.369	2.368
			4	5.648	4.560	0.966	3.239
4	11	B	1	11.157	9.112	1.910	1.882
			2	7.177	4.986	2.647	1.098
			3	5.991	4.867	2.263	1.370
			4	5.374	4.189	1.858	0.843
			5	6.328	4.715	2.778	0.446
4	12	B	1	11.270	6.604	2.961	2.100
			2	10.166	5.720	4.768	1.787
			3	10.166	5.720	4.768	1.787
4	112	A	1	8.971	9.828	3.340	2.730
			2	9.457	8.704	2.964	2.798
			3	7.959	6.847	2.537	1.165
			4	6.419	5.066	2.229	1.585
			5	6.419	5.066	2.229	1.585
4	113	A	1	11.355	3.841	3.944	2.640
			2	10.871	3.121	3.341	1.753
			3	8.048	2.146	1.486	1.100
			4	6.763	2.352	2.683	1.129
			5	6.678	1.751	2.083	1.191
4	114	A	1	14.860	6.208	5.007	3.095
			2	13.308	6.519	5.281	3.089
			3	11.623	5.541	3.795	2.615
			4	8.891	5.283	3.257	1.536
			5	5.598	4.916	2.670	1.187
4	13	B	1	5.988	4.434	1.618	0.875
			2	14.927	7.316	4.580	3.339
			3	12.838	5.624	4.174	2.982
			4	6.363	3.839	1.745	0.929
			5	16.186	9.454	5.432	3.760

Table 13.2 (cont.)

Center	Patient	Treatment	Week	HAMD factors 1	2	3	4
4	14	B	1	11.777	9.858	5.138	2.577
			2	11.570	7.199	5.852	2.363
			3	9.558	6.179	5.382	2.663
			4	8.008	5.128	4.694	1.935
			5	7.648	5.050	4.111	1.363
4	15	B	1	8.927	8.462	2.039	1.915
			2	8.330	7.694	1.587	1.717
			3	6.968	6.011	2.324	1.562
			4	6.042	4.030	1.511	0.942
			5	5.370	4.438	1.676	0.685
4	115	A	1	10.612	8.456	4.323	2.863
			2	9.630	7.644	4.125	1.992
			3	8.573	6.587	3.423	1.708
4	116	A	1	7.813	9.713	4.978	2.869
			2	7.813	9.713	4.978	2.869
4	117	A	1	14.781	8.431	4.144	3.950
			2	13.575	8.217	3.736	4.296
			3	11.297	6.158	3.141	2.663
			4	10.041	4.848	2.490	1.391
			5	6.774	4.708	1.041	2.117
4	1	B	1	14.734	7.753	5.824	2.520
			2	13.058	5.774	5.129	2.088
			3	8.165	4.737	2.125	1.171
			4	6.178	4.679	1.145	1.304
			5	11.385	5.404	3.596	0.716
4	2	B	1	10.623	8.858	5.018	2.858
			2	10.250	9.184	5.575	2.930
			3	10.250	9.184	5.575	2.930
4	3	B	1	11.724	6.612	4.107	2.199
			2	10.666	6.245	5.047	2.232
			3	10.278	7.276	5.328	2.583
			4	14.544	9.508	5.884	2.862
			5	8.191	5.854	3.411	1.121
4	4	B	1	8.976	8.309	4.976	1.435
			2	7.177	6.403	5.705	2.408
			3	7.177	6.403	5.705	2.408
4	5	B	1	10.216	8.567	4.343	2.071
			2	8.311	6.616	3.137	2.557
			3	8.311	6.616	3.137	2.557
			4	8.311	6.616	3.137	2.557

Table 13.2 (cont.)

				HAMD factors			
Center	Patient	Treatment	Week	1	2	3	4
4	6	B	1	9.077	8.661	4.051	2.558
			2	8.248	7.313	4.644	2.284
			3	7.542	6.435	4.216	2.668
4	7	B	1	14.099	8.818	4.185	2.735
			2	10.707	8.149	3.630	2.368
			3	8.185	6.220	1.718	1.218
			4	5.963	5.215	1.504	1.617
			5	10.175	7.441	3.017	2.110
4	8	B	1	13.042	11.671	4.055	2.932
			2	8.655	9.123	3.551	2.112
			3	6.392	6.537	2.336	2.310
			4	5.173	4.665	1.106	2.283
			5	4.061	3.453	1.044	1.242

In spite of the high degree of standardization established for the Hamilton Depression Scale and the stability of the four factors, there are often observable differences between raters. Because of this, the protocol required that each patient always be evaluated by the same rater. In this study, all the patients at center number 20 were evaluated by the same psychiatrist. At center number 4, one psychiatrist evaluated 20 of the patients. A colleague evaluated the other 16.

13.2. The Expected Results

This was a randomized controlled trial comparing two effective treatments. A major theme of this book is that it is not enough to describe the null hypothesis of "no effect" when designing an RCT. The trial has to start with an expected difference between treatments. If no difference is expected, then there is no reason to run the trial, since nothing is expected to be learned.

In this study, the two drugs have distinctly different pharmacological profiles in animal studies. The study was designed to determine whether a difference could be detected in humans. If such a difference exists, then the study was also designed to describe that difference and to propose possible differences in patient treatment based on presenting symptoms.

We can think of the four factors of the Hamilton Depression Scale as measuring four distinctly different aspects of clinical depression. The baseline values of these four factors describe the patient with respect to those aspects.

We can expect a patient with high values on factors I and II and low values on factors III and IV, for instance, to be different in some way from a patient with low values on factors I and II and high values on factors III and IV. If the treatments differ in their efficacy, we might expect that the degree or nature of "response" will differ between treatments for different baseline patterns.

If the treatments differ, then the amount of change on each of the factors should also differ between treatments. That is, we should be able to describe the differential effect in terms of the four uncorrelated factors, with a statement like,

Treatment A is more effective in reducing factor II (cognitive disturbance), and treatment B is more effective in reducing factor IV (sleep disturbance).

Finally, the fact that there are two centers (and three psychiatrists) doing the evaluation requires that we consider the possibility that there are differences in perceptions of disease that are due more to the rater than to differences between patients.

Thus, in order to construct a powerful restricted test, we need to direct the test against an alternative hypothesis where

(1) the treatments differ in response, as a function of the factor;
(2) the baseline balance of factors will influence the response; and
(3) there will be an effect that is due to center.

We cannot anticipate whether the differences in (1) are "in favor" of one treatment or another. So the alternative hypothesis has to include both possibilities. This means that the significance test will be "two-sided" in some sense. But, that does not mean that we have to settle for a general test that includes a large class of alternatives that do not make medical sense.

13.3. Constructing an Overall Powerful Significance Test

If we had only one factor to consider, then there is a standard method of analysis that adjusts for (2)—baseline values—and (3)—center differences—in the previous section. This is an analysis of covariance, blocked on center. That is, we let

$$Y_i = \text{measure of effect for } i\text{th patient}$$

then

$$\begin{aligned} Y_i = {} & \text{overall mean} + \text{center effect} + \text{treatment effect} \\ & + B \times (\text{baseline value}) + \text{random error} \end{aligned}$$

is a parsimonious mathematical model of what might be expected. This model assumes that the effect is linearly related to the baseline value and that the linear slope is the same for both treatments. It also assumes that there is no treatment by center interaction, that is, no effect over and above the three components described that is due to some peculiar way in which one of the centers or its patients develop a difference in response.

If we use the standard normal theory analysis of covariance, then we are also assuming that the variance of the random error is the same, regardless of treatment, and that the random error has a Gaussian, or at least a symmetric, distribution.

In this case, these seem to be safe assumptions. The factors of the Hamilton Depression Scale have been shown to be stable in three ways:

(a) The weights derived on different patient populations tend to be the same.
(b) The factors appear to have a Gaussian distribution, both when sample populations are examined and by invoking the the central limit theorem (since each is a sum of individual items).
(c) The variances across patients and the variances of differences within patient tend to be the same from population to population.

The important consideration here is that no study is done *in vacua*. The measurements we use have been used before or have some basis for selection. This means that we have a body of information that lies outside the data accumulated in the study, and it is only prudent to use that information in the construction of a powerful restricted test.

Thus, the distributional assumptions that lie behind the use of a standard analysis of covariance are not something we are simply taking on faith. We have a body of prior information that allows us to make those assumptions. Beyond the distribution of the random error, the assumptions that describe the model (linear in baseline, consistent across treatments and centers) are not so easily disposed of. It may turn out that they are not true. However, the null hypothesis is that the treatments' effects are the same. Thus, the null hypothesis subsumes all these questionable model assumptions, and a failure of any of them implies that the null hypothesis is false.

If we increase the complexity of the alternative hypothesis model, then we lose "degrees of freedom." That is, every additional parameter added to the model requires that we "use up" some of our observations to estimate that parameter. With a total of 65 patients, we have to be careful that we do not make the model so complex that there are too few patients left to provide an adequately stable estimate of the residual variance. A significance test can be thought of as a ratio of

(observed variance about the null hypothesis) ÷

(residual variance about the full alternative hypothesis).

We use t-tests and F-tests (rather than normally distributed Z-tests) because we have to take into account the fact that the denominator of the test has to be estimated and that the estimation is itself subject to random variability. Because of this, the construction of powerful restricted tests has to balance two conflicting techniques:

(i) greater specificity of the alternative hypothesis, and
(ii) precision of the estimate of residual variance.

Where that balance occurs is part of the art of statistics. With only 65 patients available, I choose to stop with the parsimonious model described earlier.

What has been described in this section so far is the construction of a powerful test for a single factor. We must yet consider how to combine such tests across all four factors. But first there is the problem of early dropouts to consider.

13.4. Dropouts

The subjects of a randomized controlled clinical trial are sick human beings. It is the primary duty of the investigator to treat their illnesses as best she or he can. If a patient is not responding to treatment, then there is a moral obligation to drop the patient from the study and seek alternative treatment. But, in the analysis of the study, the dropouts cannot be ignored, since the fact that they were removed from the study tells us something about the efficacy of the treatment.

In psychotherapeutic trials (like this one) or in any area where there is a high placebo response, it is a serious mistake to restrict analysis to only those patients who complete the full protocol. This can be seen in a comparison of placebo and active treatment. The only patients who continue to the end in the placebo arm are, by definition, those patients who have responded to placebo. Thus, the percentage of "responders" seen at the end of the study tends to be the same for all treatments. While it is possible that the mean change (the degree of "response") will differ, the numerical value of that difference has to be much less than if we could have kept the "nonresponders" in the study to the end.

Several techniques have been developed for handling dropouts. One method is to fit a linear response to all the observed values for a given patient and to compare patients with respect to the rate of response or with respect to the value of the measurement that would be predicted by that linear response at the end of the treatment period. This has the advantage that it uses "all" the data, all the intermediate values taken every two weeks in this study. It has the disadvantage that it often exaggerates the negative "response" for patients who drop out early, and the projected end-of-study value is sometimes outside the range of the measurement being analyzed.

Another technique is sometimes called the "last observation carried forward" or the "baseline-final" difference. The measure of effect on a given patient is

$$\text{last observed value} - \text{baseline value}.$$

In practice, I have found that both methods (linear slope and baseline-final) usually produce similar results. When there are a large number of intermediate observations with many missing values between the baseline and the final, it sometimes turns out that the linear slopes will have smaller within-patient variances, which increases power. In this study, with only four post-baseline observations, there does not seem to be much to be gained. We will, however, return to the intermediate observations when we seek to refine the estimates of response differences.

Whichever technique is chosen, it can be seen that we can now use all but three of the patients. The three patients for whom we have only baseline values have to be discarded from analysis unless we wish to interpolate some "response" based on the overall average "response" for that treatment group. Techniques do exist for imputing missing values in an incomplete multivariate normal vector (see Morrison [1973]). If there were many such patients, it might be worth invoking them. However, with only three patients involved, I would just drop them from the record. If the conclusions of the statistical analysis are so fragile that they would be modified by the loss of three patients, then we can hardly claim to have derived useful conclusions.

13.5. The One Overall Significance Test

A clinically reasonable alternative hypothesis (leading to an analysis of covariance blocked on clinic) has been constructed for a single factor. We now need to combine across four factors, addressing the expected alternative that the treatments may differ in response with respect to factor. To do this, we can take advantage of some mathematical theory. We know from previous work that the four factors are uncorrelated. Differences (final-baseline) are also uncorrelated. The two observed variables in the model, the difference and the baseline, are uncorrelated across factors.

The analysis of covariance provides a numerator and denominator that are used to construct an F-test of the null hypothesis. These appear in the standard ANCOVA tables (see Table 13.3) as

$$\text{numerator} = \text{mean square for treatment},$$

$$\text{denominator} = \text{mean square for residual}.$$

Under the null hypothesis, the two have the same expectation (so their ratio will tend to be randomly distributed about 1.0) and are statistically independent.

The theory of the F-distribution only requires that we take the ratio of two independently distributed random variables with chi square distribu-

Table 13.3. Analysis of Covariance Tables: Traditional Layout

Source	*d* of *f*	Mean square	*F*-statistic
Factor I			
Treatment	1	49.954	6.29
Center	1	1.828	0.23
Covariate	1	227.854	28.69
Residual	55	7.942	
Factor II			
Treatment	1	9.075	2.61
Center	1	26.041	7.48
Covariate	1	68.614	19.72
Residual	55	3.48	
Factor III			
Treatment	1	13.667	10.2
Center	1	0.479	0.36
Covariate	1	31.413	23.24
Residual	55	1.34	
Factor IV			
Treatment	1	0.392	0.55
Center	1	0.458	0.64
Covariate	1	14.905	20.98
Residual	55	0.71	

tions. The numerator of each of the four F-tests is distributed as a chi square with one degree of freedom. The denominator of each of the four F-tests is distributed as a chi square with 55 degrees of freedom. The fact that the factors are uncorrelated means that each of the numerators are independent of each other (and so, too, the denominators), and so the sum of the numerators is distributed as a chi square with 4 degrees of freedom, and the sum of the denominators is distributed as a chi square with $4 \times 55 = 220$ degrees of freedom.

Each of the mean squares for treatment is a squared deviation, and so represents a "two-sided" test, and the sum of these will be sensitive to deviations in either direction (in favor of treatment A or treatment B). Had this been a comparison between active treatment and placebo, where clinical considerations indicate that the only reasonable alternatives are one-sided, then we would have taken the square root of each of these mean squares, given it the sign of the treatment difference, summed those one-sided comparisons, and divided by the square root of the sum of the denominators (adjusted for differing sample sizes). The result would have been a one-sided t-test with 220 degrees of freedom. However, this study was between two active treatments, and the questions posed deal with differences that can go in either direction.

Table 13.4. Adjusted* Mean Scores from Analysis of Covariance

	Adjusted means	
Factor	Drug A	Drug B
I	−3.319	−2.099
II	−1.745	−1.177
III	−1.176	−0.381
IV	−0.342	−0.332

* Effects predicted by the analysis of covariance model if all patients had the same baseline values. This common value is set at the average baseline across all patients.

The sum of the mean squares for treatment is

$$49.954 + 9.075 + 13.667 + 0.392 = 73.088.$$

The sum of the mean squares for residual is

$$7.942 + 3.480 + 1.340 + 0.710 = 13.473.$$

This leads to an F-test with (4,220) degrees of freedom of

$$F(4{,}220) = 5.425, \; p = 0.0003.$$

Thus, there is highly significant evidence that there was a difference in effect between the two treatments. We now have a license to hunt. Table 13.4 displays the adjusted mean effects by treatment for each factor. The relative effects can be teased out of such a table.

[At this point, the proponents of multivariate normal methods are ready to pounce. Why did I use this method (which can be described as the trace of a matrix of response) instead of the more general multivariate analysis of covariance (MANCOVA), for which we now have many exquisite computer packages? In fact, we might have gotten a similar result. However, blind use of MANCOVA continues a pernicious statistical fiction that dominates too much of the literature of RCTs. This is the fiction that the only "information" we have is what we can derive from the data in this study. MANCOVA requires, among other things, that we estimate the correlations between the factors from the 65 patient records, that we use these estimates, and, then, that we adjust the test to take into account the random uncertainty associated with estimating the correlations from a small set of data. However, all information does not come from this study. We know that the four factors are uncorrelated. We don't have to waste degrees of freedom estimating those correlations. One of the reasons I wrote this book is to point out to the medical/statistical community that "standard" methods of analysis (which assume that there are no external sources of information) are not the best methods to use.]

Table 13.5. Clusters of Patients with Similar Baseline

Cluster 1		Cluster 2		Cluster 3		Cluster 4		Cluster 5	
Drug A	Drug B	Drug A	Drug B	Drug A	Drug B	Drug A	Drug B	Drug A	Drug B
20-12	20-1	20-17	4-010	20-20	20-15	20-23	20-7	20-25	20-3
13	2	4-110	14	4-106	19	4-102	4-008	26	4-009
16	8	105	11	113	4-015	101	3	4-100	1
18	10	109	13	104	4	111	5	117	
19	11	108	12	116	2			103	
22	14	107		103				114	
24	20	112							
27	4-006								
28	7								
4-115									

Table 13.6. Two-Way Analysis of Variance: Clusters versus Treatment

Source	d of f	Mean square	F-test
Factor I			
Treatment	1	38.665	3.37
Cluster	4	36.238	0.79
Interaction	4	48.406	1.06
Residual	48	11.463	
Factor II			
Treatment	1	7.367	1.49
Cluster	4	35.984	1.83
Interaction	4	13.508	0.69
Residual	48	4.928	
Factor III			
Treatment	1	13.234	9.09
Cluster	4	24.062	4.13
Interaction	4	9.534	1.64
Residual	48	1.456	
Factor IV			
Treatment	1	0.268	0.27
Cluster	4	2.296	0.59
Interaction	4	3.772	0.96
Residual	48	0.979	

13.6. Alternative Methods of Analysis

The one overall significance test described in Section 13.5 was derived from what might be expected from treatment differences. This should always be the starting point of any analysis. However, the method described in Section 13.5 is only one of several general methods that have been discussed in earlier chapters. These data can be used to illustrate some of those other methods. In what follows, we will analyze the data with other methods, merely as illustration, keeping in mind that a method may not be optimal if there is no medically defensible model of the alternative hypothesis behind it.

13.6.1. Blocking on Baseline Characteristics to Get More Homogeneous Blocks

The baseline values for the four factors were examined with the use of a multidimensional projection program, MacSpin$_{TM}$ (see Donoho, Donoho, Romano, and Olson [1985]), and five clusters emerged. That is, there appears to be five groups of patients with similar patterns in terms of the four baseline factors. The resulting patient groupings are displayed in Table 13.5. Table 13.6 displays the two-way analyses of variance for final-baseline changes in factor 2 that result from comparing treatment effects, first by blocking on clinic, second by blocking on baseline cluster. It can be seen that the baseline clusters, by providing more homogeneous patient groups, produces a lower p-value and thus has greater power. This illustrates the general principle that we can usually increase the power by blocking patients into subgroups with similar baseline characteristics or with similar etiologies. The mean squares for the four factors produce $F_{(4,192)} = 3.162$, $p < .01$.

13.6.2. Analysis of Maximum and Dominant Symptom

Table 13.7 displays the measurements, with each of the factors now standardized

$$Y_i = (X_i - \min(i))/(\max(i) - \min(i)),$$

where

$\min(i)$ = minimum value of factor i across all observed values in the study,

$\max(i)$ = maximum value of factor i across all observed values in the study.

Ignoring the known (uncorrelated) structure of the factor analysis, we can now think of these factors as scores of different aspects of the disease. If we think of the four standardized numbers as describing a spectrum of symptoms, it is obvious that some patients have different spectrums than others and that the spectrum of symptoms tends to change across time. Two approaches to such a problem that were suggested earlier were the use of

dominant symptom = factor with the greatest standardized baseline value for that patient,

maximum symptom = factor with the greatest standardized value at a given visit for that patient.

Least squares linear slopes were computed for each patient based on the standardized factors for the sequence of values of the dominant symptom and the sequence of maximum symptom values. To illustrate, consider patient number 803, at center number 20.

The dominant "symptom" is factor 4. Over time the value goes down by more than 2/3. The linear slope is -0.151 per week. The maximum symptom, however, changes as follows:

baseline, factor 4;
week 2, factor 4;
week 4, factor 4;
week 6, factor 2; and
week 8, factor 2;

and these values have a linear slope of -0.073.

Table 13.7. Hamilton Depression Scale Factor Scores

				Normalized HAMD factors			
Center	Patient	Treatment	Week	1	2	3	4
20	1	B	1	0.312	0.305	0.275	0.250
			2	0.624	0.611	0.549	0.501
			3	0.209	0.395	0.590	0.246
			4	0.161	0.647	0.473	0.334
			5	0.161	0.647	0.473	0.334
20	2	B	1	0.289	0.312	0.371	0.221
			2	0.577	0.623	0.741	0.442
			3	0.613	0.654	0.747	0.542
			4	0.662	0.563	0.605	0.615
20	3	B	1	0.304	0.338	0.392	0.245
			2	0.608	0.676	0.785	0.491
			3	0.756	0.555	0.775	0.744
			4	0.358	0.643	0.501	0.584
			5	0.416	0.704	0.573	0.530
20	4	B	1	0.304	0.256	0.304	0.321
			2	0.607	0.511	0.608	0.642
			3	0.667	0.522	0.648	0.510
			4	0.485	0.565	0.432	0.681
			5	0.578	0.484	0.624	0.651
20	5	B	1	0.232	0.305	0.180	0.219
20	6	B	1	0.304	0.254	0.395	0.445
			2	0.609	0.509	0.791	0.890
			3	0.376	0.455	0.526	0.580
			4	0.326	0.383	0.450	0.529
			5	0.122	0.573	0.543	0.282
20	7	B	1	0.317	0.285	0.333	0.348
			2	0.634	0.570	0.666	0.697
20	8	B	1	0.339	0.285	0.277	0.244
			2	0.667	0.570	0.553	0.487
20	9	B	1	0.359	0.284	0.317	0.280
			2	0.718	0.569	0.635	0.559
			3	0.423	0.555	0.376	0.379
20	10	B	1	0.273	0.256	0.276	0.203
			2	0.546	0.511	0.552	0.406
			3	0.040	0.000	0.000	0.003
			4	0.040	0.000	0.000	0.003
			5	0.040	0.000	0.000	0.003
20	11	B	1	0.300	0.319	0.257	0.286
			2	0.600	0.638	0.514	0.571

Table 13.7 (cont.)

Center	Patient	Treatment	Week	Normalized HAMD factors			
				1	2	3	4
			3	0.728	0.695	0.686	0.516
			4	0.722	0.655	0.700	0.591
			5	0.371	0.465	0.557	0.479
20	12	A	1	0.399	0.263	0.259	0.288
			2	0.798	0.526	0.517	0.575
			3	0.567	0.611	0.581	0.501
			4	0.516	0.550	0.554	0.572
			5	0.305	0.440	0.303	0.623
20	13	A	1	0.343	0.280	0.278	0.298
			2	0.686	0.560	0.556	0.597
			3	0.653	0.583	0.636	0.704
20	14	B	1	0.371	0.289	0.339	0.266
			2	0.742	0.579	0.677	0.531
			3	0.665	0.586	0.527	0.497
			4	0.486	0.432	0.491	0.353
			5	0.509	0.457	0.602	0.426
20	15	A	1	0.310	0.318	0.384	0.360
20	16	A	1	0.322	0.224	0.461	0.233
			2	0.644	0.449	0.921	0.466
			3	0.557	0.618	0.660	0.619
			4	0.605	0.558	0.470	0.505
			5	0.624	0.527	0.588	0.441
20	17	A	1	0.330	0.350	0.386	0.233
			2	0.659	0.700	0.772	0.466
			3	0.467	0.605	0.658	0.694
			4	0.367	0.563	0.553	0.451
20	18	A	1	0.327	0.391	0.326	0.260
			2	0.655	0.782	0.653	0.520
			3	0.548	0.627	0.599	0.659
			4	0.335	0.521	0.585	0.436
20	19	A	1	0.321	0.308	0.333	0.266
			2	0.642	0.616	0.665	0.532
			3	0.599	0.569	0.578	0.368
			4	0.673	0.586	0.572	0.514
20	20	B	1	0.279	0.293	0.320	0.293
			2	0.559	0.587	0.640	0.587
			3	0.638	0.219	0.374	0.579
			4	0.370	0.635	0.485	0.509
20	21	A	1	0.332	0.308	0.432	0.297

Table 13.7 (cont.)

Center	Patient	Treatment	Week	Normalized HAMD factors			
				1	2	3	4
20	22	A	1	0.359	0.315	0.336	0.220
			2	0.718	0.629	0.671	0.440
			3	0.651	0.601	0.637	0.547
			4	0.415	0.600	0.471	0.546
20	23	A	1	0.342	0.306	0.321	0.305
			2	0.684	0.613	0.642	0.610
			3	0.699	0.578	0.728	0.545
			4	0.663	0.412	0.389	0.683
			5	0.579	0.595	0.607	0.491
20	24	A	1	0.277	0.288	0.281	0.269
			2	0.554	0.576	0.561	0.537
			3	0.644	0.558	0.548	0.424
			4	0.477	0.618	0.426	0.390
			5	0.482	0.602	0.407	0.363
20	25	A	1	0.307	0.337	0.360	0.293
			2	0.614	0.674	0.719	0.587
			3	0.614	0.674	0.719	0.587
			4	0.639	0.560	0.474	0.529
			5	0.708	0.664	0.679	0.789
20	26	A	1	0.383	0.327	0.418	0.319
			2	0.766	0.655	0.837	0.638
			3	0.683	0.580	0.700	0.653
			4	0.475	0.722	0.474	0.398
			5	0.475	0.722	0.474	0.398
20	27	A	1	0.264	0.312	0.257	0.222
			2	0.528	0.624	0.514	0.443
20	28	A	1	0.250	0.323	0.287	0.246
			2	0.500	0.647	0.573	0.492
			3	0.293	0.556	0.559	0.701
			4	0.271	0.455	0.617	0.433
			5	0.335	0.516	0.603	0.471
20	29	A	1	0.272	0.274	0.323	0.252
			2	0.543	0.547	0.646	0.503
			3	0.528	0.624	0.514	0.443
			4	0.663	0.529	0.666	0.811
			5	0.356	0.479	0.410	0.371
4	100	A	1	0.449	0.401	0.495	0.258
			2	0.897	0.802	0.990	0.516
			3	0.461	0.424	0.336	0.129
			4	0.394	0.357	0.397	0.025
			5	0.158	0.351	0.272	0.000

Table 13.7 (cont.)

Center	Patient	Treatment	Week	Normalized HAMD factors 1	2	3	4
4	101	A	1	0.267	0.414	0.386	0.254
			2	0.535	0.828	0.773	0.508
			3	0.427	0.459	0.544	0.336
			4	0.258	0.327	0.137	0.181
			5	0.095	0.289	0.094	0.301
4	102	A	1	0.348	0.362	0.500	0.448
			2	0.697	0.724	1.000	0.895
			3	0.549	0.569	0.609	0.452
			4	0.197	0.304	0.326	0.307
			5	0.146	0.348	0.871	0.487
4	103	A	1	0.366	0.342	0.298	0.147
			2	0.733	0.684	0.596	0.294
			3	0.085	0.311	0.329	0.478
4	104	A	1	0.164	0.276	0.127	0.164
			2	0.327	0.552	0.254	0.329
			3	0.199	0.655	0.614	0.220
			4	0.212	0.689	0.633	0.183
			5	0.446	0.709	0.448	0.239
4	105	A	1	0.234	0.435	0.301	0.193
			2	0.468	0.871	0.602	0.385
4	106	A	1	0.215	0.267	0.362	0.290
			2	0.429	0.533	0.724	0.581
			3	0.429	0.533	0.724	0.581
			4	0.157	0.417	0.445	0.510
			5	0.106	0.357	0.419	0.581
4	107	A	1	0.377	0.437	0.285	0.254
			2	0.754	0.874	0.569	0.508
			3	0.536	0.787	0.512	0.599
			4	0.363	0.512	0.344	0.495
			5	0.133	0.332	0.226	0.047
4	108	A	1	0.340	0.369	0.191	0.292
			2	0.680	0.738	0.383	0.583
			3	0.680	0.738	0.383	0.583
4	109	A	1	0.448	0.381	0.287	0.204
			2	0.895	0.763	0.574	0.408
			3	0.495	0.671	0.419	0.399
4	9	B	1	0.361	0.270	0.369	0.175
			2	0.721	0.539	0.738	0.349
			3	0.545	0.457	0.601	0.229
			4	0.395	0.363	0.483	0.063

Table 13.7 (cont.)

				Normalized HAMD factors			
Center	Patient	Treatment	Week	1	2	3	4
4	10	B	1	0.306	0.416	0.383	0.224
			2	0.611	0.831	0.765	0.449
			3	0.493	0.650	0.881	0.424
4	110	A	1	0.377	0.386	0.455	0.226
			2	0.754	0.772	0.910	0.452
			3	0.272	0.429	0.450	0.575
			4	0.129	0.315	0.256	0.423
			5	0.103	0.376	0.362	0.200
4	111	A	1	0.449	0.338	0.290	0.284
			2	0.898	0.675	0.581	0.569
			3	0.517	0.530	0.423	0.393
			4	0.262	0.344	0.334	0.507
4	11	B	1	0.293	0.380	0.128	0.191
			2	0.585	0.760	0.257	0.383
			3	0.257	0.374	0.380	0.182
			4	0.159	0.363	0.316	0.252
			5	0.108	0.299	0.248	0.117
4	12	B	1	0.297	0.263	0.216	0.219
			2	0.595	0.525	0.432	0.439
			3	0.504	0.443	0.734	0.358
4	112	A	1	0.202	0.414	0.248	0.300
			2	0.405	0.827	0.495	0.600
			3	0.445	0.722	0.433	0.617
			4	0.321	0.548	0.362	0.199
			5	0.194	0.381	0.310	0.307
4	113	A	1	0.301	0.133	0.298	0.288
			2	0.602	0.267	0.596	0.577
			3	0.562	0.199	0.496	0.350
			4	0.329	0.108	0.186	0.183
			5	0.223	0.127	0.386	0.190
4	114	A	1	0.445	0.244	0.387	0.346
			2	0.891	0.488	0.774	0.693
			3	0.763	0.517	0.819	0.691
			4	0.624	0.426	0.571	0.570
			5	0.398	0.402	0.482	0.294
4	13	B	1	0.079	0.161	0.104	0.063
			2	0.159	0.322	0.208	0.125
			3	0.896	0.592	0.702	0.755
			4	0.724	0.434	0.635	0.664
			5	0.190	0.266	0.229	0.139

Table 13.7 (cont.)

				Normalized HAMD factors			
Center	Patient	Treatment	Week	1	2	3	4
4	1 4	B	1	0.318	0.415	0.398	0.280
			2	0.636	0.830	0.795	0.560
			3	0.619	0.581	0.915	0.506
			4	0.453	0.486	0.836	0.582
			5	0.326	0.387	0.721	0.396
4	15	B	1	0.201	0.350	0.139	0.196
			2	0.401	0.699	0.278	0.391
			3	0.352	0.627	0.203	0.341
			4	0.240	0.470	0.326	0.301
			5	0.163	0.284	0.190	0.142
4	115	A	1	0.270	0.349	0.330	0.317
			2	0.540	0.699	0.659	0.634
			3	0.459	0.623	0.626	0.411
4	116	A	1	0.155	0.408	0.384	0.318
			2	0.309	0.817	0.769	0.635
4	117	A	1	0.442	0.348	0.315	0.456
			2	0.884	0.697	0.630	0.912
			3	0.785	0.676	0.562	1.000
			4	0.597	0.484	0.462	0.582
			5	0.493	0.361	0.354	0.257
4	1	B	1	0.440	0.317	0.455	0.273
			2	0.880	0.633	0.910	0.546
			3	0.742	0.448	0.794	0.435
			4	0.338	0.351	0.293	0.201
			5	0.175	0.345	0.129	0.235
4	2	B	1	0.271	0.368	0.388	0.316
			2	0.541	0.737	0.775	0.632
			3	0.510	0.767	0.868	0.651
4	3	B	1	0.316	0.263	0.312	0.232
			2	0.632	0.526	0.623	0.464
			3	0.545	0.492	0.780	0.472
			4	0.513	0.588	0.827	0.562
			5	0.865	0.797	0.920	0.633
4	4	B	1	0.203	0.343	0.384	0.134
			2	0.405	0.685	0.768	0.268
			3	0.257	0.507	0.890	0.517
4	5	B	1	0.254	0.355	0.331	0.216
			2	0.508	0.709	0.663	0.431
			3	0.351	0.527	0.462	0.555
			4	0.351	0.527	0.462	0.555

Table 13.7 (cont.)

Center	Patient	Treatment	Week	Normalized HAMD factors			
				1	2	3	4
4	6	B	1	0.207	0.359	0.307	0.278
			2	0.414	0.718	0.614	0.556
			3	0.345	0.592	0.713	0.486
4	7	B	1	0.414	0.366	0.318	0.300
			2	0.828	0.733	0.636	0.601
			3	0.548	0.670	0.544	0.507
			4	0.340	0.489	0.225	0.213
			5	0.157	0.395	0.189	0.315
4	8	B	1	0.370	0.500	0.307	0.326
			2	0.741	1.000	0.615	0.651
			3	0.379	0.761	0.531	0.442
			4	0.192	0.519	0.328	0.492
			5	0.092	0.344	0.123	0.485

Table 13.8. Patient 803, Center 20

Factor	Baseline	Week 2	Week 4	Week 6	Week 8
1	0.609	0.376	0.326	0.122	0.122
2	0.509	0.455	0.383	0.573	0.573
3	0.791	0.526	0.450	0.543	0.543
4	0.890	0.580	0.529	0.282	0.282

The dominant symptom is the most severe presenting symptom and allows us to track the course of disease in terms of presenting symptoms. Use of the maximum symptom allows us to examine an upper "envelope" of disease, knowing that all symptoms are less than or equal to the maximum one.

Table 13.9 displays the analysis of variance tables (treatment by clinic) for the two slopes, dominant symptom, and maximum symptom.

13.7. Life Beyond Significance

Coming back to the restricted test of Section 13.5, the one constructed from reasonable clinical expectations, the analysis indicated a highly significant difference between treatments ($p = 0.0003$). This tells us that there is some sort of a "signal" in the study. The goal of the remaining analysis should be to identify the nature of that "signal" and to provide a measure of the uncertainty associated with those findings.

Table 13.9. Analyses of Variance on Slopes of Dominant Maximum Symptom

Source	d of f	Mean square	F-statistic	Significance level
Dominant symptom:	1			
Treatment	1	0.0367	5.39	0.024
Center	1	0.0143	2.1	0.153
(treatment) × (center)	1	0.0027	0.39	0.532
Residual	55	0.0068		
Maximum symptom:				
Treatment	1	0.0212	4.1	0.045
Center	1	0.0288	5.71	0.02
(treatment) × (center)	1	0.0096	1.9	0.173
Residual	55	0.005		

In general, we will be using two tools. One of them is Neyman's confidence interval. If we provide a numerical answer to some question, the confidence interval provides us with the extreme values of that answer that would just barely be rejected by a significance test. For instance, once we have established that there is a difference in response pattern associated with the set of four factors, a reasonable question is, What is the mean difference with respect to baseline-final changes in factor I?

13.7.1. Interval Estimates of the Mean

The analysis of covariance on changes in factor I produced estimates of mean change:

Treatment A: -3.319 ($n = 32$),
Treatment B: -2.099 ($n = 27$), and
Mean square for residual: 7.942.

There are sophisticated methods for deriving confidence bounds on treatment differences, using the algorithms of the analysis of variance. Each method leads to a slightly different set of bounds, and there are serious definitional problems about what theoretical parameter or linear combinations of parameters is being estimated (see Searle [1972]). However. one of the points made in this book is that there is no good philosophical definition of the meaning of probability in terms of "real life" and the best we can do is identify those things that are highly probable and those that have probability of around 50 percent. Thus the slight differences in coverage probability or endpoint values that result from use of one model or another are of no practical value.

With this in mind, it should be adequate to compute a rough estimate of the ends of the confidence intervals. This can be done by estimating the standard error of the mean difference as

$$MSE(1/32 + 1/27) = 0.542$$

and adding and subtracting some multiple of this to the observed mean difference. Thus, for an approximately 95 percent confidence interval we take

$$2.099 - 3.319 + 2\,\mathrm{sqrt}(0.542) = -1.220 \pm 1.472, \quad \text{or} \quad (-2.69, 0.2).$$

An approximate 50 percent confidence interval is

$$2.099 - 3.319 \pm 0.674\,\mathrm{sqrt}(0.542) = -1.220 \pm 0.496, \quad \text{or} \quad (-1.716, -0.724).$$

From this, we can say that we are "quite sure" that the effect of Treatment A is no greater than 2.64 units more than the effect of Treatment B. Or we can say that there is a 50:50 chance that the difference is in favor of Treatment A, with the difference lying between 1.7 and 0.7 units. For those whose personal probabilities allow them to consider probabilities between 50 percent and 95 percent, a 75 percent confidence interval is $(-2.019, -0.421)$.

This, of course, begs the question of what we mean by the units of the factors. A confidence interval on some underlying mean has to be constructed on units of measurement that have some clinical meaning, or the answer becomes an empty exercise in statistics.

There may be some who can accept vague ideas like being "quite sure" or a 50:50 chance, but to whom the statements about "effect" are too vague. They might ask what we mean by "effect." Since we are describing parameters of a probability distribution, it is possible to define "effect" a little better. Suppose that this RCT will be used to propose some aspect of general medical practice and that the treatments will henceforth be used on a large number of similar patients. We can then say that we are quite sure that the observed average difference in change on factor 1 for this very large future population will lie between -2.6 and 0.2 and there is a 50 percent chance that It will be between -1.7 and -0.7.

The vague ideas of "quite sure" and "50:50" can be made mathematically exact by inserting the problem into a Bayesian paradigm. Now we start with some prior idea of the mean difference in "effect" between treatment A and treatment B. Suppose, for the sake of argument, the medical scientist has prior belief in the relative efficacy of treatment A versus treatment B and she says that she is "quite sure" that the mean difference in effect on factor 1 lies between -4 and -1. Her prior belief can now be modeled as if the mean difference were normally distributed with the parameters

$$\text{underlying mean} = ([-4] + [-1])/2 = -2.5,$$

$$2 \text{ standard deviations} = ([-2.5] - [-4]) = 1.5,$$

$$\text{underlying standard deviation} = 0.75, \quad \text{or}$$

$$\text{underlying variance} = 0.5625.$$

If we observe an average difference of X with an estimated standard error of S, then the posterior distribution of the mean difference will have

$$\text{underlying mean} = (0.5625X + (-2.5)S^2)/(0.5625 + S^2),$$

$$\text{underlying variance} = (0.5625S^2)/(0.5625 + S^2).$$

In this case, where $X = -1.22$ and $S^2 = 0.504$, the posterior distribution has

$$\text{underlying mean} = -1.825,$$

$$\text{underlying variance} = 0.266,$$

$$\text{underlying standard deviation} = 0.516.$$

Posterior probability regions on the mean differences are

$$95\%: (-2.67, -0.98) = (-1.825 \pm 1.645 \times 0.516),$$

$$50\%: (-2.20, -1.50) = (-1.825 \pm 0.674 \times 0.516).$$

These are tighter bounds than those produced by traditional confidence intervals, but this is because they reflect a degree of prior belief. Had the medical scientist indicated much more uncertainty, the posterior bounds would have been wider. In fact, had she indicated that she believed that the mean difference could range from -100 to 100, or any other very wide interval (leading to a very large underlying variance for the prior), it is clear, from the formula for computing the posterior mean and variance, that the Bayesian posterior bounds would have been very close to the traditional confidence interval bounds.

13.7.2. Medically Meaningful Interval Estimates

This whole exercise of computing interval estimates of the mean difference in effect assumes that there is some clear medical interpretation for the numerical value of change on a given factor score. This is obviously not true. The factors of the Hamilton Depression Scale have little clinical meaning in terms of absolute value. However, there is meaning in their relative value. A patient with relatively high baseline scores on one factor and not on others represents a particular presentation of symptoms. And, so, a reasonable medical question one might ask of the data is, Is treatment A better than treatment B for patients whose most prominent presenting symptoms lead to high values on factor 2?

The word *better* can be interpreted in two ways (when it comes to modeling the question in order to get a numerical answer). One treatment is *better* than another if the probability that a patient will improve is greater on the first. Or, a treatment is *better* than another if the average change score is greater on it. We examined interval estimates of mean changes in the previous paragraphs. Let us consider numerical answers fashioned around the probability of improving.

The probability of improvement, when comparing two treatments, can be viewed in two different ways. Let

$$X = \text{the response of a patient to treatment A},$$

$$Y = \text{the response of the same patient to treatment B}.$$

Suppose there are fixed levels of "response" such that a patient responds to treatment A if

$$X > C, \quad \text{for some fixed number } C,$$

and similarly to treatment B (if $Y > C$). To fix ideas, let C represent a 50 percent decrease from baseline. Using Table 13.7 (the standardized values of the factor scores), we can see that there are only six patients whose baselines have factor 4 as the most prominent factor:

Center	Patient number	Treatment	Baseline	Final
4	106	A	0.581	0.581
4	112	A	0.600	0.307
4	117	A	0.912	0.443
20	801	B	0.632	0.319
20	803	B	0.890	0.282
20	805	B	0.697	0.657

These are not very many, and we would expect that the resulting confidence bounds will be quite wide. In fact, for this set of patients, treatment is confounded with center, so any difference that we find may be due to either treatment or clinic or both. A far more precise answer can be computed if we look at changes in factor 3. However, I leave that as an exercise for the reader. The results for factor 3 are so neat that the reader should have the pleasure of discovering them.

When we compare probabilities of events between two treatments, the "natural parameter" is the odds ratio:

$$pA(1 - pB)/[pB(1 - pA)], \quad \text{where} \quad pA = \text{Prob}\{\text{event for treatment A}\}$$
$$\text{and} \quad pB = \text{Prob}\{\text{event for treatment B}\}.$$

This is a natural parameter because it is the parameter that has to be used when computing power for the "standard" tests like the Fisher–Irwin exact test. If we observe

$$X = \text{number of patients with events on treatment A},$$

$$Nx = \text{number of patients on treatment A},$$

$$Y = \text{number of patients with events on treatment B},$$

$$Ny = \text{number of patients on treatment B},$$

then an estimator of the odds is

$$R = X(Ny - Y)/[Y(Nx - X)],$$

and the approximate variance of the natural logarithm of R is

$$1/X + 1/(Nx - X) + 1/Y + 1/(Ny - Y).$$

When the sample is small, as in this case, there is a high probability that one of the four values $(X, Nx - X, Y, Ny - Y)$ will be zero. So the estimator is often modified by adding 0.5 to all values. In this case,

$$X = 1.5,$$
$$Nx - X = 2.5,$$
$$Y = 1.5,$$
$$Ny - Y = 2.5.$$

$$R = 1.0,$$
$$\log(R) = 0,$$
$$\mathrm{var}(\log(R)) = 1/X + 1/(Nx - X) + 1/Y + 1/(Ny - Y) = 2.983,$$

standard deviation = S.D. = 1.727.

$$\log(R) \pm 2\mathrm{S.D.} = 0 \pm 3.454,$$
$$\log(R) \pm 0.674\mathrm{S.D.} = 0 \pm 1.164.$$

Using antilogs, this converts to approximate confidence intervals:

98 percent: R lies within (0.0316, 31.6),

50 percent: R lies within (0.312, 3.203).

The problem with computing bounds on odds ratios is that it is difficult to convert these to clinically meaningful values. In some very vague sense, an odds ratio of 31:6 means that the probability of response on treatment A is around 5 times greater than the probability of response on treatment B.

Most people think in terms of difference is probabilities, rather than ratios of odds. So, it is more politic to present confidence bounds on

$$pA - pB = \mathrm{Prob}\{\text{response on A}\} - \mathrm{Prob}\{\text{response on B}\}.$$

There are more exact estimates of confidence bounds on differences than the following one. In fact, there are mathematical statisticians who have almost made a profession out of this problem. But if we consider confidence bounds to be rough approximations of vague ideas, then the following should be good enough.

The parameters pA and pB can be estimated by X/Nx and Y/Ny. Or to avoid zeros in small samples by

$$\hat{p}A = (X + 0.5)/(Nx + 0.5),$$
$$\hat{p}B = (Y + 0.5)/(Ny + 0.5).$$

If the two probabilities are nearly the same, then an overall estimate of their common value is

$$\hat{p}S = (X + Y + 0.5)/(Nx + Ny + 0.5),$$

leading to an estimate of the variance of the difference, $\hat{p}A - \hat{p}B$, of the form

$$\hat{\text{var}} = \hat{p}S(1 - \hat{p}S)(1/Nx + 1/Ny).$$

These can now be used to compute confidence bounds.

In the case at hand,

$$\hat{p}S = 2.5/6.5 = 0.385,$$

$$\hat{\text{var}} = 0.158$$

and confidence bounds are

95 percent: $0 \pm 2\,\text{sqrt}(0.158) = 0 \pm 0.795$,
50 percent: $0 \pm 0.674\,\text{sqrt}(0.158) = 0 \pm 0.268$.

There is a rough Bayesian approach, which treats the difference in probabilities as if they were normally distributed. Thus, suppose the clinician starts with a prior belief that treatment A is superior, in this respect, to treatment B and that the difference in probability of response lies between

$$0.1 \quad \text{and} \quad 0.9.$$

This yields a prior of

$$\text{underlying mean} = 0.5,$$

$$\text{underlying variance} = [(0.9 - 0.1)/4]^2 = 0.04.$$

We observed

$$\text{mean} = 0,$$

$$\text{variance} = 0.158,$$

leading to a posterior distribution with

$$\text{underlying mean} = 0.399,$$

$$\text{underlying variance} = .0319.$$

The posterior 95 percent probability region

$$(0.041, 0.756)$$

is strongly influenced by the prior belief.

If the prior belief had been much wider, say -1.0 to 1.0, then the prior would have

$$\text{underlying mean} = 0.0,$$

$$\text{underlying variance} = 0.25,$$

and the posterior would have

$$\text{underlying mean} = 0.0,$$

$$\text{underlying variance} = .097,$$

and the posterior 95 percent probability region would be

$$(-.622, 0.622),$$

much closer to the 95 percent confidence bounds of $(-0.795, 0.795)$.

13.7.3. Interval Estimates Based on Nonparametric Tests

As indicated earlier, the question of whether treatment A is more effective than treatment B can be addressed by considering the theoretical random variables

$$X = \text{response of a given patient to treatment A},$$

$$Y = \text{response of the same patient to treatment B}.$$

It is obvious that we cannot put the same patient on both treatments, so we have to infer the relationship between these two theoretical responses from what happened to patients who were randomly assigned to A or B. From these we can estimate the parameter

$$PP = \text{Prob}\{X < Y\}.$$

If the two treatments are equivalent (under this measure), then PP is equal to 0.5. If A is superior to B, then PP is less than 0.5, and vice versa. This is a very natural parameter to think in terms of. It has nothing to do with the scale of measurement yet it uses more information about the response than simply indicating whether the observed measurement was greater than some fixed value. It also turns out that this is the natural parameter of the Wilcoxon rank sum test. In fact, an estimator of PP can be derived directly from the Wilcoxon test. If

$$W = \text{the sum of the ranks of the patients on treatment A},$$

$$Nx = \text{number of patients on treatment A},$$

$$Ny = \text{number of patients on treatment B},$$

then

$$\widehat{PP} = (W - Nx(Nx + 1)/2)/Nx\,Ny$$

is a consistent, unbiased, minimum-variance, asymptotically normal estimator of PP. Its exact variance is easily computed as

$$\text{Var} = (Nx + Ny + 1)/(12Nx\,Ny).$$

In the case at hand the changes final-baseline can be ordered

Treatment A	Rank	Treatment B	Rank
0.000	1	0.040	2
0.293	3	0.313	4
0.469	5	0.608	6

So the sum of the ranks for treatment A is 9 ($= 1 + 3 + 5$), the estimate of PP is

$$\widehat{PP} = (9 - 3(4)/2)/9 = 0.5,$$

and its exact variance is

$$\text{var} = (3 + 3 + 1)/108 = 0.0648.$$

Using normal approximations, the confidence bounds are

95%: $(-0.009, 1.009) = 0.5 \pm 0.509$,
50%: $(0.328, 0.672) = 0.5 \pm 0.172$.

A literal interpretation of the 95 percent confidence bounds makes no sense since probabilities cannot be less than 0 nor greater than 1.0, but what these confidence bounds mean, in the vague sense proposed in this book, is that we cannot be sure of anything about $\text{Prob}\{X < Y\}$.

As before, the fact that $\widehat{PP}$ is asymptotically normally distributed means that we can apply a Bayesian prior and use the same formulas as were used earlier to compute posterior distributions that describe the measure of belief held by the individual scientist.

13.8. Further Exploration

This discussion of Bayesian posterior regions has skipped a number of mathematical niceties. The observed sample variances have been treated as if they were, in fact, the true variances. Efron and Morris [1962, 1963] have shown how to modify the analysis to take the random noise in these estimates into account. The conjugate prior distribution for a binomial is the beta distribution, and a more accurate translation of prior belief might have been to model the two probabilities, pA and pB, as two independent beta-variables, so the posterior distribution of their differences would have been the convolution of two betas. But all of these are neat complications that can be easily put into a black box and turned over to the computer to calculate. What I have attempted to do here is to show is that one can actually calculate numerical values to associate with measures of belief.

If we stay within the Bayesian paradigm, then there is no problem taking subsets of patients (such as those whose most prominent symptoms are reflected in factor 4). The sequence

$$\text{prior} \rightarrow \text{observed data} \rightarrow \text{posterior}$$

has no restrictions on how or where the observed data are taken from. There is no need to maintain some overall probability of error or to be sure that all patients randomized to treatment are in the analysis. In this book, I have advocated that we pay close attention to these problems when constructing the one big overall significance test that enables us to know whether there is any "signal" in the midst of the random noise. Once we know there is a "signal," however, it does not much matter how we shovel the random noise out of the way—at least this is so in the Bayesian paradigm.

If we compute confidence intervals without reference to Bayesian priors, then we are faced with the unsolved philosophical problem of what is meant by the "coverage" of such an interval. When the statistician computes a 95 percent confidence interval, the medical scientist has a right to ask, "95 percent of what?" As indicated in the early chapters of this book, the standard academic answer, based on frequentist theory, is not satisfactory. It carries within it the seeds of serious inconsistencies, and its very careful statement about confidence intervals that will be calculated in the future provides no useful information to the practicing scientist who must interpret the one particular study at hand.

I have, instead, advocated that we use the tools of confidence intervals to compute a "smear" of uncertainty to put around our estimates of effect. I cannot guarantee that the "smear" has any particular probabilistic meaning. We may calculate it with 95 percent or 50 percent probability statements, but these are only convenient cut-points that enable us to make a calculation. If we use a large number (like 95 percent) for one type of interval and a small number (like 50 percent) for the other, we come close to meeting the vague ideas that most people have about things that are "sure" and things that are "50:50." The confidence intervals calculations guarantee us two things

The 95 *percent "smear" will be larger than the* 50 *percent "smear."*
The greater the number of patients involved the smaller the "smear."

This sort of knowledge is usually sufficient for most uses. When the European explorers of the 16th and 17th centuries set out for the New World, they needed to know the distance across the Atlantic only to a sufficient degree of accuracy that would allow them to take along enough provisions. And when they looked at the stars in an attempt to find out where they were, it was sufficient to distinguish between being one day or one week away from landfall. This degree of vagueness, however, would not be adequate for a cruise missile. To launch these ground-hugging robot bombs against a specific target, the armed forces need to know the exact location of the target, and the missile needs to plot its course with a degree of accuracy that would have been inconceivable to Adrian Block, the 17th-century explorer.

I claim that the needs of medical science that can be supplied by randomized controlled trials demand a degree of accuracy closer to that needed by the 16th to 17th-century explorers than to that of a modern cruise missile—at least when it comes to computing probabilities and statistical estimates of effect.

The reader is left to examine the rest of the data in Table 13.1. We know from the overall significance test that there are differences between treatment. A careful look at that data will show some of them. Look, for instance, at the question of time to response. If you restrict attention to the 26 patients whose final values were less than 50 percent of baseline for at least one factor, you will find a difference in time to response that can be estimated with relatively little "smear." The relative consistency of changes from baseline across the four factors will turn out to be dependent upon center. If you look at changes in factor 3 as a function of baseline you will find other treatment differences with possible implications for therapeutics. As long as you keep computing the 95 percent confidence bounds or Bayesian posterior probability regions, you can avoid being trapped by Anscombe's will-o-the-wisps.

Good luck, and remember that statistics should be the handmaiden of medical research ... and not its jailer.

References

In addition to articles and books specifically referred to in Chapters 1 to 13, this annotated bibliography directs the reader's attention to further discussions of many of the topics touched on in the text.

Abramowitz, M., and Stegan, I.A., Eds. (1964) *Handbook of Mathematical Functions.* Applied Math Series, vol. 55. National Bureau of Standards.
A compendium of mathematical functions, formulas, tables, and approximations that covers almost all an applied mathematician needs.

Anscombe, F.J. (1948) The transformation of Poisson, binomial and negative binomial data. *Biometrika 35*, 246–254.
One of the first papers that approached transformations from a robust point of view.

Anscombe, F.J. (1957) Dependence of the fiducial argument on the sampling rule. *Biometrika 44*, 464–469.
This is one of the earlier papers in the literature that reveals some of the fundamental inconsistencies that occur with the Neyman–Pearson formulation.

Anscombe, F.J. (1960) Examination of Residuals. In *Proceedings of the 4th Berkeley Symposium on Mathematical Statistics and Probability* (Neyman, Ed.), vol. I, 1–36.
A commonsense view of that aspect of data analysis in which the model is compared to the data.

Anscombe, F.J. (1963) Tests of goodness of fit. *J. Royal Statistical Society* (*B*), *25*, 81–94.
Compares Fisherian, Neyman–Pearson, and Bayesian ideas.

Anscombe, F.J. (1985) Comments on "A coherent view of statistical inference" by G.A. Barnard. Statistical and Technical Report Series, Dept. of Statistics and Actuarial Science, Univ. of Waterloo.
Makes the point that clinical studies usually test treatments that can be expected to have an effect, so the statistical methods should be optimized for the situation where the null hypothesis is probably not true.

Anscombe, F.J. (1990) The summarizing of clinical experiments by significance levels. *Statistics in Medicine*, *9*, 703–708.
Expands on the ideas in Anscombe (1985) and points out that the best use of

statistics in analyzing RCTs is not to test the null hypothesis but to make inferences about the alternative.

Anscombe, F.J., and Tukey, J.W. (1963) The examination and analysis of residuals. *Technometrics*, *5*, 141–160.
Takes up the ideas in Anscombe (1960).

Armitage, P. (1955) Tests for linear trends in proportions and frequencies. *Biometrics*, *11*, 375–386.
The Armitage–Cochran test.

Arvesen, J.N., and Layard, M.W.J. (1971) Asymptotically robust tests in unbalanced variance component models. Purdue University Dept. of Statistics, Mimeograph Series #263.

Arvesen, J.N., and Salsburg, D.S. (1973) Approximate tests and confidence intervals using the jackknife. In *Perspectives in Biometry* (Elashoff, Ed.) Academic Press, New York.
Both papers show how transformations of the data can be used to produce symmetric pseudovariates and improve the behavior of the jackknife.

Bahadur, R.R., and Savage, L.J. (1956) The nonexistence of certain statistical procedures in nonparametric problems. *Annals of Mathematical Statistics*, *27*, 1115–1122.
Technically difficult to read, this paper describes classes of probability distributions for which no test of hypothesis can be constructed that will detect differences among members of the class.

Barlow, R.E., Bartholomew, D.J., Bremner, J.M., and Brunk, H.D. (1972) *Statistical Inference Under Order Restrictions*, John Wiley & Sons, New York.
Brunk estimators are described in Chapter 2. Bartholomew's test is described in Chapter 3.

Barnard, G.A. (1985) A coherent view of statistical inference. *Statistics and Technical Report Series*, Dept. of Statistics and Actuarial Science, Univ. of Waterloo.
Barnard is a major figure in the development of mathematical statistics, who, starting in the late 1930s, made significant contributions to the theories that lie behind the use of "standard" tests. This paper is part of later work, in which he attempts to find a general overall theory of statistical inference, which would have none of the contradictions of the Neyman–Pearson model.

Barnard, G.A. (1990) Must clinical trials be large? The interpretation of p-values and the combination of test results. *Statistics in Medicine*, *9*, 601–614.
Criticizes the rigid use of 5 percent and 1 percent significance tests and recommends alternatives to strict Neyman–Pearson testing.

Begg, C.B. (1990) Suspended judgment: Significance tests of covariate imbalance in clinical trials. *Controlled Clinical Trials*, *11*, 223–225.
Discusses the problem of possible "imbalance" at baseline between randomized treatment groups, finds that the practice of first testing for imbalance and then "adjusting" for it if imbalance is found is potentially misleading.

Behrens, W.U. (1964) Comparison of means of normal distributions with different variances. *Biometrics*, *20*, 66.
A survey paper that covers the methods used to adjust the two-sample t-test for differing variances.

Berger, J. (1983) The frequentist viewpoint and conditioning. In *Proceedings of the Berkeley Conference in Honor of Jerzy Neyman and Jack Kiefer*, (LeCam and Olshen, Ed.), vol. 1, Wadsworth Publishing Co., Monterey, Calif.
A very lucid description of the fundamental inconsistencies that have been found with the frequentist theory of probability and its application in the Neyman–Pearson formulation. This paper describes Kiefer's attempts to modify the theory and points out where the attempts fail.

Berger, J.O., and Sellke, (1987) Testing a point null hypothesis, the irreconcilability of p-values and evidence. *J. Amer. Stat. Assn.*, *82*, 112–139 (with discussion).

One of two papers (see also Casella and Berger (1987)) that appeared side by side with discussion. This paper shows a number of situations where tail p-values make no sense. The companion paper attempts to link p-values and Bayesian posterior probabilities and shows only limited success.

Birnbaum, A. (1962) On the foundations of statistical inference. *J. Amer. Stat. Assn.*, *57*, 269–306.

Birnbaum, A. (1977) The Neyman–Pearson theory as decision theory and as inference theory: With a criticism of the Lindley-Savage argument for Bayesian theory. *Synthese*, *36*, 19–49.

These two papers represent the "best" effort of one of the deepest thinkers in mathematical statistics to justify frequentist probability theory.

Box, G.E.P. (1980) Sampling and Bayes' inference in scientific modeling and robustness. *J. Royal Statistical Society* (*A*), *143*, part 4, 383–430 (with discussion).

Box has made major contributions to several branches of statistics, including time series, response surfaces, and Bayesian analysis. In this paper (amplified in the accompanying discussion), he lays out the general problems of frequentist interpretations (called "sampling" here) and the solutions that can be found in Bayesian interpretations. The paper is lucid, and most of it can be read and understood by someone not familiar with the technical notation used.

Box, G.E.P., and Cox, D.R. (1964) An analysis of transformations. *J. Royal Statistical Soc.* (*A*), *26*, 211–253.

The development of power transformations where the power that best normalizes the data can be estimated directly from the data.

Breslow, N. (1990) Biostatistics and Bayes. *Statistical Science*, *5*, 267–298 (with discussion).

A carefully developed full discussion of how Bayesian techniques have been or could be used in the analysis of clinical data.

Brown, L.D. (1990) An ancillarity paradox which appears in multiple linear regression (1985 Wald Memorial Lectures). *Annals of Statistics*, *18*, 471–538 (with discussion).

Technically difficult to read, this paper shows how a Bayesian definition of probability is necessary if the results of a single study are to be extrapolated to different populations of patients.

Brownie, C., Boos, D.D., and Hughes-Oliver, J. (1990) Modifying the t and ANOVA F tests when treatment is expected to increase variability relative to controls. *Biometrics*, *46*, 259–266.

A simple alternative to the "standard" methods that takes advantage of what might be expected if the null hypothesis were not true.

Canner, P.L. (1983) Comment on "Statistical inference from clinical trials: Choosing the right p-value." *Controlled Clinical Trials*, *4*, 13–18.

Advocates use of Bayesian and likelihood inferences in clinical trials.

Casella, G., and Berger, R.L. (1987) Reconciling Bayesian and frequentist evidence in a one-sided testing problem. *J. Amer. Stat. Assn.*, *82*, 106–111 (with discussion 123–139).

One of two papers (see also Berger and Sellke (1987) that appeared side by side. This paper tries to identify situations where p-values can be interpreted in terms of Bayesian posterior distributions. The other paper shows situations where p-values make no sense.

Chinchilli, V.M., and Sen, P.K. (1981) Multivariate linear rank statistics and the union-intersection principle for hypothesis testing under restricted alternatives. *Sankya*, *43B*, 135–151.

Provides a general method for constructing nonparametric and restricted statistical tests in a multivariate setting.

Cohen, L.J. (1989) *An Introduction to the Philosophy of Induction and Probability.* Clarendon Press, Oxford.

A comprehensive discussion of the philosophical problems involved in attempts to use probability statements to develop scientific theories. Cohen discusses several solutions to the problem and proposes one of his own, based on formal modal logic.

Conover, W.J. (1980) *Practical Non-parametric Statistics*, 2d ed. John Wiley & Sons, New York.

Conover, W.J., and Salsburg, D.S. (1988) Locally most powerful tests for detecting treatment effects when only a subset of patients can be expected to "respond" to treatment. *Biometrics*, *44*, 198–196.
Describes a nonparametric restricted test that has proved quite useful in the analysis of clinical trials.

Copas, J.B. (1972) Empirical Bayes methods and the repeated use of a standard. *Biometrika*, *59*, 349–360.
Example of Robbins' empirical Bayes procedures, when the analyst has more information available than can be found in the study at hand.

Cornfield, J. (1976) Recent methodological contributions to clinical trials. *American J. of Epidemiology*, *104*, 408–421.
Cornfield was the first statistician on the Framingham study and developed the now widely used method of logistic regression. He had extensive experience working at NIH in the design and analysis of clinical trials. His untimely death cut short the work described in this paper, where he advocates the use of Bayesian likelihood and utility functions in the analysis of clinical studies rather than the Neyman–Pearson formulation.

Cox, D.R. (1958) Some problems connected with statistical inference. *Annals of Math. Stat.*, *29*, 357–372.

Cox, D.R. (1977) The role of significance tests. *Scand. Journal of Statistics*, *4*, 49–70.
In this paper Cox presents a full-blown theory of significance testing, based on the pragmatic Fisher approach.

Dallal, G.E. (1988) Pitman: A FORTRAN program for exact randomization tests. *Computers and Biomedical Research*, *21*, 9–15.

David, F.N. (1947) A χ^2 'smooth' test for goodness of fit. *Biometrika*, *34*, 299–310.

Dempster, A.P. (1968) Upper and lower probabilities generated by a random closed interval." *Annals of Math. Stat.* *39*, 957–966.
This is an alternative definition of probability as applied to the results of scientific studies. It is usually referenced in any paper that describes foundational theory, but the definition and its attendant methods are seldom used. In spite of its lack of use, the definition offers many advantages that might prove useful in the interpretation of clinical trials.

DiCiccio, T.J., and Romano, J.P. (1985) A review of bootstrap confidence intervals. *J. Royal Statistical Soc.* (*B*), *50*, 338–370 (with discussion).
A very readable review of the bootstrap and various modifications designed to produce "better" confidence intervals. The discussion, as is usual with the Royal Statistical Society, provides excellent insights into how many prominent statisticians have used the bootstrap.

Dimear, G.T., and Layard, W.M.J. (1973) A Monte Carlo study of asymptotically robust tests for correlation coefficients. *Biometrika*, *60*, 551–558.
Investigation of the effect of different transformations on behavior of the jackknife.

Donoho, H.W., Donoho, D.L., Gasko, M., and Olson, C.W. (1985) *MACSPIN Graphical Data Analysis Software*. D^2 Software, Austin, Tex.
Software for the Macintosh computer, which uses the ideas of projection-pursuit.

Eden, T., and Yates, F. (1933) On the validity of Fisher's Z test when applied to an actual example of non-normal data. *J. Agricultural Science*, *23*, 7–17.
Ostensibly a description of the robustness of what we now call analysis of variance, this paper provides some useful insights into what Fisher and his coworkers meant by significance testing. Eden and Yates were both early associates of Fisher's.

Edwards, A.W.F. (1972) *Likelihood*, Cambridge University Press, Cambridge.

An easily understood and well-written exposition of the likelihood principle and associated techniques. Edwards advocates that we do away with formal significance tests (since, as he points out, their "meaning" is not clear) and work with values of the likelihood function to determine confidence regions for well-defined parameters.

Efron, B. (1969) Student's t-test under symmetry conditions. *J. Amer. Stat. Assn.*, *64*, 1278–1284.

Theoretical proof that the one-sample t-test is robust to nonnormality of a particular kind.

Efron, B. (1982) *The Jackknife, the Bootstrap, and Other Resampling Plans.* SIAM, Philadelphia.

Efron B. (1987) Better bootstrap confidence intervals. *J. Amer. Stat. Assn.*, *14*, 1431–1452 (with discussion).

Efron, B., and Morris, C. (1962) Limiting the risk of Bayes and empirical Bayes estimators, part 1. J. Amer. Stat. Assn., *67*, 130–144.

Efron, B., and Morris, C. (1963) Limiting the risk of Bayes and empirical Bayes estimators, part II. *J. Amer. Stat. Assn.*, *68*, 117–125.

These two papers establish the maximum likelihood methods for estimating parameters in an empirical Bayesian setting.

Efron, B., and Tibshirani, R. (1986) Bootstrap methods for standard errors, confidence intervals, and other methods of statistical accuracy. *Statistical Science*, *1*, 54–77.

Efron developed a general method of statistical inference based on the straightforward use of the empirical distribution function of the observed data, which he called the "boostrap." These papers describe the bootstrap and its uses.

Feinstein, A. (1971) How do we measure "safety" and "efficacy"? Clinical Biostatistics IX. *Clinical Pharm. Therap.*, *12*, 544–569.

Feinstein A. (1973) The role of randomization in sampling, testing, allocation, and credulous idolatry (part 2)—Clinical biostatistics XXIII, *Clinical Pharm. Therap.*, *14*, 898–916.

Feinstein has questioned the "standard" statistical methodology from the standpoint of the medical scientist. In the second paper, he advocates the use of permutation tests.

Fisher, R.A. (1921) Studies in crop variation I, An examination of the yield of dressed grain Broadbalk. *Journal of Agricultural Science*, *11*, 107–135 (Paper 15 in *Collected Papers of R.A. Fisher*, the University of Adelaid, Australia, 1971).

A good example of Fisher as the statistician analyzing data. In this paper he uses significance tests in the fashion proposed in this book.

Fisher, R.A. (1926) The arrangement of field experiments. *Journal of the Ministry of Agriculture of Great Britain*, *33*, 505–513 (Paper 48 in *Collected Papers*).

Shows how randomized assignment is essential to the use of significance tests and deplores the use of systematic arrangements.

Fisher, R.A. (1929) The statistical method in psychical research. In *Proc. of the Society for Psychical Research, vol. 39*, 189–192 (Paper 79 in *Collected Papers*).

A fairly complete exposition of what Fisher meant by significance testing and the use of a 5 percent p-value.

Fisher, R.A. (1935) Statistical tests. *Nature*, *136*, 474 (Paper 127 in *Collected Papers*).

A vehement denunciation of the idea of "accepting the null hypothesis" or Neyman's type II error.

Fisher, R.A. (1937) Professor Karl Pearson and the method of moments. *Annals of Eugenics*, *7*, 303–318 (Paper 149 in *Collected Works*).

In the midst of what is mostly petty criticism of Pearson's work, Fisher discusses the usefulness and interpretation of the statistical analysis of data.

Fisher, R.A. (1951) *The Design of Experiments.* Hafner Publishing Co., New York.

Section 9, pp. 17–21, covers randomization and permutation tests. Section 61, pp. 185–188, discusses problems resulting from multiplicity of tests and claims that one can use several different tests on the same data, as long as each test questions a different aspect of the null hypothesis.

Fisher, R.A. (1955) Statistical methods and scientific induction. *J. Royal Statistical Soc. (B)*, *17*, 69–78 (Paper 261 in *Collected Works*).

Fisher, R.A. (1959) *Statistical Methods and Scientific Inference.* Oliver and Boyd, Edinburgh and London.
In the previous paper and in a more expanded fashion in this book, Fisher attacks the Neyman–Pearson formulation of hypothesis testing and articulates his own view of the relationship between statistical methods and science. His major criticism of the N-P formulation is that it does not describe the thought processes that go into scientific development and that the whole concept of type I and type II errors makes no sense in the development of scientific inference.

Fisher, R.A. (1970) *Statistical Methods for Research Workers*, 14th ed. Oliver and Boyd, Edinburgh and London.
This is Fisher's classic "cookbook." This book went through 14 editions, the first in 1925, as he added to and modified the techniques. The book is filled with the general sense of pragmatic usefulness that dominated Fisher's own approach to statistical analysis. Section 21.1 describes the method of combining independent significance tests by adding the logs of the *p*-values.

Fisz, M. (1963) *Probability Theory and Mathematical Statistics*, 3d ed. John Wiley & Sons, New York.
Chapter 11, "An outline of the theory of runs."

Fix, E., Hodges, J.L., and Lehmann, E.L. (1959) The restricted Chi square test. In *Probability and Statistics, the Harald Cramer Volume* (Ulf Grenander, ed.), John Wiley & Sons, New York.
Although Neyman developed the method of restricted chi square tests, there is no single paper by Neyman that describes the technique in its full range of possibility. This paper, by Neyman's colleagues, does.

Freeman, M . F., and Tukey, J .W. (1950) Transformations related to the angular and the square root. *Ann. of Math Stat.*, *28*, 602–632.
Modifications to the standard transformations of the Poisson and binomial to account for contaminated distributions.

Friedman, J.H., and Rafksy, L.C. (1983) Graph-theoretic measures of multivariate association and prediction. *Annals of Stat.*, *11* 377–391.
Proposes a class of test statistics for the problem when the vector of measures on each patient is larger than the number of patients. The test statistics are based on construction of graph "trees" connecting the individual points.

Gans, D.J. (1981) Corrected and extended tables for Tukey's quick test. *Technometrics*, *23*, 193–195.

Gart, J.J. (1971) The comparison of proportions, a review of significance tests, confidence intervals, and adjustments for stratification. *Review of the Int. Stat. Inst.*, *39*, 148–169.
A solid review article on the topic of comparing two binomials.

Gosset, W.S. (1931) The Lanarkshire milk experiment. *Biometrika*, *23*, 398 (appears as paper #16 in "*Student's*" *Collected Papers*, (Pearson and Wishart, eds.), University Press, Cambridge, 1942.
The classic example of a randomized controlled clinical trial with a fundamental flaw and a foolish finding.

Hajek, J. (1968) Asymptotic normality of simple linear ranks statistics under alternatives. *Annals of Math. Stat.*, *37*, 325–346.
The theoretical paper that underlies the development of locally most powerful restricted nonparametric tests. Using Hajek's methods, it is possible to construct a "best" test statistic for any class of alternatives that can be identified.

Hajek, J., and Sidak, Z. (1967) *Theory of Rank Tests.* Academic Press, New York

A classic book that reduces the entire field of nonparametric tests to a simple formulation involving the relative ranks of observations.

Henze, N. (1988) A multivariate two-sample test based on the number of nearest neighbor type coincidences. *Annals of Statistics, 16*, 772–783.
A nonparametric multivariate test that uses the power of the modern computer and appears to be much more powerful than the "standard" normal theory-based tests.

Hinkley, D.V. (1988) Bootstrap methods. *J. Royal Statistical Soc. (B), 50*, 321–337.
A very readable description of the bootstrap and its uses.

Hollander, M., and Wolfe, D.A. (1973) *Nonparametric Statistical Methods*, John Wiley & Sons, New York.
An excellent compendium of nonparametric methods, with a good selection of restricted test procedures.

Hui, S.I, and Berger, J.O. (1983) Empirical Bayes estimation in longitudinal studies. *J. Amer. Stat. Assn., 78*, 753–760.

Hurwitz, R.A. (1991) Personal communication regarding work in progress.

Johnson, R.A., Verrill, S., and Moore, D.H. II (1988) Two sample rank tests for detecting changes that occur in a small proportion of the treated population. *Biometrics, 43*, 641–655.
Describes a group of nonparametric restricted tests for a class of alternatives similar to the ones described in the paper by Conover and Salsburg.

Kahneman, D., Slovic, P., and Tversky, A. (1982) *Judgement Under Uncertainty: Heuristics and Biases.* Cambridge University Press, Cambridge.
Contains a description of experiments that attempted to elucidate coherent personal probabilities from individuals.

Keynes, J.M. (1921) *A Treatise on Probability.* Macmillan, London.

Kiefer, J. (1976) Admissibility of conditional confidence procedures. *Annals of Statistics, 4*, 836–865.
Kiefer's attempt to modify the Neyman–Pearson formulation in order to solve its theoretical problems.

Lachin, J.M. (1988) Properties of randomization in clinical trials. *Controlled Clinical Trials, 9*, 287–311.
This is a set of four articles describing methods for randomizing patients to treatment and the statistical theories that lie behind randomization. Written for the nonspecialist, they contain the best and most complete description of the theory and practice that I have seen in any medical or statistical journal.

Laird, N.M, and Louis, J.A. (1987) Empirical Bayes confidence intervals based on Bootstrap samples. *J. Amer. Stat. Assn., 82*, 739–757. (with discussion).
A how-to-do-it paper for computing Bayesian confidence intervals via the bootstrap.

Lehmann, E.L. (1959) *Testing Statistical Hypotheses.* John Wiley & Sons, New York.
The most complete exposition of the Neyman–Pearson formulation and all its ramifications.

Lindley, D.V. (1990) The present position in Bayesian statistics (The 1988 Wald Memorial Lectures). *Statistical Science, 5*, 44–89.
Lindley, a leading advocate of Bayesian methods, presents a very readable and complete description of these ideas.

Loeve, M. (1968) *Probability Theory*, 3d ed. D. Van Nostrand Co., Princeton, N.J.
Glivenko-Cantelli lemma on page 20.

Mantel, N. (1963) Chi square tests with one degree of freedom; Extensions of the Mantel-Haenszel procedure. *J. Amer. Stat. Assn., 58*, 690–700.
A full discussion of the Mantel–Haenszel method.

Mau, J. (1988) A generalization of a non-parametric test for stochastically ordered distributions to censored survival data. *J. Royal Statistical Society (B), 50*, 403–412.
A significance test that can handle the situation where the alternative hypothesis involves ordering and the data are censored. This is an example of the many

"nonstandard" statistical methods that are available in the statistical literature once the analyst starts looking for restricted tests.

Mehta, C.R., Patel, N.R., and Senchaudhur, P. (1988a) Exact and Monte Carlo methods for computing non-parametric significance tests. *SUGI*, *13*, 1065–1070.

Mehta, C.R., Patel, N.R., and Wei, L.J. (1988b) Constructing exact significance tests with restricted randomization rules. *Biometrika*, *75*, 295–302.
These are two of a large number of papers published by Mehta and colleagues, in which they exploit optimum search routines discovered earlier by Mehta to generate significance levels for permutation tests. Many of these tests have been incorporated into proprietary software developed by Mehta and associates under the brandname STATXACT.

Miller, R.G. Jr. (1968) Jackknifing variances. *Ann. Math. Stat.*, *39*, 567–582.
A jackknife-based test for equality of variances.

Morris, C.N. (1983) Parametric empirical Bayes inference: Theory and applications. *J. Amer. Stat. Assn.*, *78*, 47–59.
A full discussion of Morris' approach to empirical Bayes, where the hyperparameters are imbedded in the likelihood function and are estimated from the data.

Morrison, D.F. (1967) Multivariate Statistics. McGraw Hill, New York.

Morrison, D.F. (1973) A test for equality of means of correlated variates with missing data on one response. *Biometrika*, *60*, 101–105.
A modern computer-intensive technique for handling missing data.

Mosteller, F., and Youtz, C. (1990) Quantifying probabilistic expressions. *Statistical Science*, *5*, 2–34.
An examination of the "practical" meaning of probabilistic phrases like "highly probable."

Neyman, J. (1934) On the two aspects of the representative method. *J. Royal Statistical Society*, *97*, 558–625 (with discussion).
This is the first appearance of Neyman's confidence intervals. The development, a Bayesian one, is the one I used in this book.

Neyman, J. (1935a) Sur la verification des hypotheses statistiques composees. *Bulletin de la Societe Mathematique de France*, *63*, 246–266.
This is the last paper Neyman wrote on the subject of hypothesis testing. It is a survey paper, hitting the high points of the development described in the three previous papers. It contains the statement that "unhappily" conditions required for what we now call uniformly most powerful test seldom occur. Neyman never attacked the N-P formulation, but in his later papers he avoided use of it.

Neyman, J. (1935b) On the problem of confidence intervals. *Annals of Math. Stat.*, *6*, 111–116.
This later description of confidence intervals does not contain the earlier Bayesian development and provides the current "standard" interpretation.

Neyman, J. (1949) Contribution to the theory of the χ^2 test. In *Proceedings of the 1st Berkeley Symposium on Mathematical Statistics and Probability*, 239–273.
Neyman's description of restricted chi-square tests.

Neyman, J., and Pearson, E.S. (1928) On the use and interpretation of certain test criteria. *Biometrika*, *20a*, Part I, 175–240; Part II, 263–294.

Neyman, J., and Pearson, E.S. (1933a) The testing of statistical hypotheses in relation to probabilities a priori. In *Proceedings of the Cambridge Philosophical Society*, vol. 29, 492–510.

Neyman, J., and Pearson, E.S. (1933b) On the problem of the most efficient tests of statistical hypotheses. *Philosophical Transactions* (*A*), *231*, 289–337.
These are the three classic papers in which Neyman and Pearson developed and described the formulation of hypothesis testing that now bears their name. Current terminology is due to Lehmann, but the basic concepts and the mathematical theory behind them are laid out in these papers.

Noether, G.E. (1967) *Elements of Nonparametric Statistics.* John Wiley & Sons, New York.
The theoretical foundations of nonparametric tests, along with a discussion of the effects of departures from assumptions.
O'Brien, P.C. (1984) Procedures for comparing samples with multiple endpoints. *Biometrics, 40,* 1679–1087.
A method for combining relative ranks across several measures to produce a single overall significance test of the type advocated in this book.
O'Hagan, A. (1988) *Probability, Method, and Measurement.* Chapman and Hall, London.
Personal Bayes's methods and proofs.
Pearson, E.S. (1962) Some thoughts on statistical inference. *Annals of Math. Stat., 33,* 394–403.
The other member of the Neyman–Pearson formulation weighs in 30 years later with some serious questions about blind use of that formulation.
Posten, H.O. (1978) The robustness of the two sample t-test over the Pearson system. *J. Statis. Comput. Simul., 6,* 295–311.
Monte Carlo study showing the robustness of p-values for a two-sample t-test across a range of distributions.
Robbins, H. (1964) The empirical Bayes approach to statistics. In *Proceedings of the 3d Berkeley Symposium on Mathematical Statistics and Probability* (Neyman, Ed.), vol. 1, 157–164.
Robbins's view of what empirical Bayes is all about.
Salsburg, D. (1981) Development of statistical analysis for single dose bronchodilators. *Controlled Clinical Trials, 2,* 305–317.
Describes the statistical analysis of a class of clinical trials, where the test statistics were derived from clinically meaningful expectations of effect.
Salsburg, D. (1989) Use of restricted significance tests in clinical trials: Beyond the one- versus two-tailed controversy. *Controlled Clinical Trials, 10,* 71–82.
Salsburg, D. (1990) Hypothesis versus significance testing for controlled clinical trials: A dialogue. *Statistics in Medicine, 9,* 201–211.
Two earlier papers discussing the main ideas of this book.
Savage, L.J. (1954) *The Foundations of Statistics.* John Wiley & Sons, New York.
Savage's major work on the theory of probability as it can be applied to the science of life, ending up with the finding that the only sensible meaning of probability is in terms of personal probability.
Savage, L.J. (1961) The foundations of statistics reconsidered. In *Proceedings of the 4th Berkeley Symposium on Mathematical Statistics and Probability.* (Neyman, ed.), vol. I, 579–586.
Second thoughts and a response to critics of his 1954 book.
Savage, L.J. (1967) Difficulties in the theory of personal probability. *Philosophy of Science, 34,* 305–310.
Further development of the concept of personal probability.
Searle, S. (1972) *Linear Models.* John Wiley & Sons, New York.
Has a detailed discussion of exactly what linear combination of means are estimated within the framework of various unbalanced analyses of variance.
Severini, T.A. (1991) On the relationship between Bayesian and non-Bayesian interval estimates. *J. Royal Statistical Society (B), 53,* 611–618.
In this book I have glossed over the fact that frequentist confidence intervals do not exactly equal posterior Bayes predictive intervals. In this paper, Severini established conditions under which the two are very close. In general, the two are close when the probability distribution of the data belongs to the exponential family (which includes most of the distributions discussed in elementary statistics courses) and when the prior distribution, the scientists's prior belief about the parameter being estimated, is diffuse and relatively uninformative.

Shafer, G. (1990) The unity and diversity of probability. *Statistical Science*, *5*, 435–462.
An easily read discussion of the various interpretations of probability that have appeared in the statistical and scientific literature.

Sheffe, H. (1959) *The Analysis of Variance*. John Wiley & Sons, New York.
Chapter 10 deals with robustness.

Siegal, S., and Tukey, J.W. (1960) A nonparametric sum of ranks procedure for relative spread in unpaired samples. *J. Amer. Stat. Assn.*, *55*, 429–445.
Nonparametric test for equality of variances.

Smith, C.A.B. (1961) Consistency in statistical inference and decision. *J. Royal Statistical Society* (*B*), *23*, 1–37.
Another view of statistics as based on personal probability.

Thompson, G.L. (1991) A unified approach to rank tests for multivariate and repeated measures designs. *J. Amer. Stat. Assn.*, *86*, 410–419.
This paper presents a general method for using Hajek transformations of ranks to construct powerful test statistics against well-defined alternatives within the framework of even the most complicated designs.

Tiao, G.C., and Box, G.E.P. (1973) Some comments on Bayes' estimators. *American Statistician*, *27*(2), 12–14.
A readable exposition of the basic Bayesian ideas.

Tukey, J.W. (1957) On the comparative anatomy of transformations. *Annals of Mathematical Statistics*, *28*, 602–632.
An overall theory of transformations.

Tukey, J.W. (1962) The future of data analysis. *Annals of Mathematical Statistics*, *33*, 1–67.
Discusses the use of split samples.

Tukey, J.W. (1977) Some thoughts on clinical trials, especially problems of multiplicity. *Science*, *198*, 679–684.
Tukey is the great original thinker of statistical theory during the last half of the 20th century. He has revolutionized almost every aspect of statistical theory and practice. This provides the reader with still another approach to the analysis of clinical trials.

Tukey, J. W. (1989) Remarks presented at a symposium in honor of Joseph Ciminera, Philadelphia, Pa.
Proposes a method for generating permutation tests with a smaller number of legal permutations to enumerate.

Tversky, A., and Kahneman, D. (1983) Extensional versus intuitive reasoning: The conjunction fallacy in probability judgement. *Psychological Rev.*, *90*, 293–315.
Relates the experiences of experimental psychologists in failing to elicit coherent person probabilities.

Welch, B.L. (1958) On linear combinations of several variances. *J. Amer. Stat. Assn.*, *53*, 777–790.

Wittes, J., and Wallenstein, S. (1987) The power of the mantel-Haenszel test. *J. Amer. Stat. Assn.*, *82*, 1104–1109.
Defines alternative hypotheses against which the Mantel-Haenszel–test is and is not powerful.

Index

Springer Series in Statistics

(continued from p. ii)

Salsburg: The Use of Restricted Significance Tests in Clinical Trials.
Särndal/Swensson/Wretman: Model Assisted Survey Sampling.
Seneta: Non-Negative Matrices and Markov Chains.
Shedler: Regeneration and Networks of Queues.
Siegmund: Sequential Analysis: Tests and Confidence Intervals.
Todorovic: An Introduction to Stochastic Processes and Their Applications.
Tong: The Multivariate Normal Distribution.
Vapnik: Estimation of Dependences Based on Empirical Data.
West/Harrison: Bayesian Forecasting and Dynamic Models.
Wolter: Introduction to Variance Estimation.
Yaglom: Correlation Theory of Stationary and Related Random Functions I: Basic Results.
Yaglom: Correlation Theory of Stationary and Related Random Functions II: Supplementary Notes and References.